The Alchemy of Addiction

Within this important book, Stephen J. Costello draws on Eastern philosophy, Western psychology, and wisdom traditions to offer an interpretation and answer to the multidimensional problem of addiction.

The nature of pleasure, pain, and attachment are discussed, together with stress as a key source of our suffering. Justifying and grounding the work is C. G. Jung's central insight that the solution to our disordered desires lies in cultivating a spiritual approach to life. As such, a detailed exploration of the Twelve Steps of recovery is elucidated from the threefold perspective of the philosophy of Advaita, the Enneagram system, and the Christian contemplations of Richard Rohr, John Main, and Thomas Keating, as well as St Ignatius of Loyola. The work concludes with a brief look at Platonic ethics, especially the virtue of temperance, St Benedict's spirituality of humility, and the law of *dharma* as a blueprint for purposeful non-addicted living.

This book will appeal to a wide variety of readers such as mental health professionals in the counselling and psychotherapy professions, as well as students of depth psychology and philosophy.

Stephen J. Costello is an acclaimed philosopher, depth psychologist, and Enneagram coach. He was educated at St Gerard's School, Castleknock College, and University College Dublin, where he graduated with BA, MA, and PhD degrees in philosophy. He subsequently trained first in psychoanalysis (Trinity College) and then in logotherapy and existential analysis (USA and Vienna). He is the author of sixteen books and is the founder-director of the Viktor Frankl Institute of Ireland, which offers online diploma courses and training. He leads corporate seminars and clinical workshops both nationally and internationally. His website is www.stephenjcostello.com.

'Dr Costello offers to addiction studies what Ken Wilber brought to human knowledge. His book integrates the profound teachings and wisdom of Buddhism, Hinduism, Western and Eastern philosophies, as well as the vast body of psychological and psychiatric knowledge related to addiction. In this groundbreaking work, he elucidates the pressing need to include "spirituality" as an essential component in the treatment of all addiction, ranging from alcoholism to pornography. Drawing from his extensive experience as a trained analyst, Dr Costello provides profound insights into the complex nature of addiction. He courageously challenges the prevailing approach, highlighting the pitfalls of prescribing drugs to combat primary chemical dependencies and the psychotherapeutic futility of searching for non-existent childhood causes. Instead, he convincingly shows that a spiritual solution is paramount in addressing the multifaceted problem of addiction. Not only will this enthralling book captivate those struggling with addiction, but it will also resonate with individuals concerned about their loved ones. With its potential to transform the fields of medicine, psychology, and psychotherapy, this enlightening masterpiece deserves to be required reading for all aspiring medical professionals. Brilliant, inspiring, and deeply nourishing to the soul, this page-turner offers solace and guidance, serving as a timeless resource for those seeking genuine understanding and growth.'

Dr Ian Mc Cabe, *PhD, PsyD, LLM is a Chartered Clinical Psychologist,*
Child and Adult Jungian Analyst, and the author of
Carl Jung and Alcoholics Anonymous

The Alchemy of Addiction

Carl Jung, the Enneagram, and
Contemplative Wisdom Traditions

Stephen J. Costello

Routledge
Taylor & Francis Group

LONDON AND NEW YORK

Designed cover image: The Alchemist by Thomas Wijck (1640–1677), Rijksmuseum, Dupper Wzn. Bequest, Dordrecht

First published 2025
by Routledge
4 Park Square, Milton Park, Abingdon, Oxon OX14 4RN

and by Routledge
605 Third Avenue, New York, NY 10158

Routledge is an imprint of the Taylor & Francis Group, an informa business

© 2025 Stephen J. Costello

British Library Cataloguing-in-Publication Data
A catalogue record for this book is available from the British Library

ISBN: 978-1-032-72776-9 (hbk)
ISBN: 978-1-032-72777-6 (pbk)
ISBN: 978-1-003-42257-0 (ebk)

DOI: 10.4324/9781003422570

Typeset in Times New Roman
by SPi Technologies India Pvt Ltd (Straive)

I dedicate this book to Thomas O'Connor

Contents

Acknowledgements

I would like to extend a huge thanks to my parents, Val and Johnny, for their enduring support of and interest in my work. My gratitude also goes to my friends, especially Darren Cleary, Tom O'Connor, to whom I dedicate this book, Cathal O'Keeffe, and Jack Morris. Profound appreciation also goes to Dr Ian Mc Cabe for his beautiful and extremely kind endorsement of this book, which both humbles and honours me, and for which I am so appreciative.

Introduction

This book is intended primarily for individuals and groups working with addiction and/or the Enneagram. I draw on Eastern philosophy, Western psychology, and wisdom teachings to offer an interpretation of and solution (an old alchemical word) to the problem of addiction.

Topics covered include the nature of pleasure, pain, and attachment; stress and the sources of our suffering; ego (personality) versus Self (essence); Carl Jung's cardinal insight: *spiritus contra spiritum* as a guiding principle throughout – that the solution to 'spirits' is in spirituality (after all, even the etymology of the word 'addiction' coming from the Latin *addico* suggests being given over to something in devotion), as well as alchemical research; our threefold energy; a detailed exploration of the Twelve Steps of Recovery, including a chapter on meditation, drawing on (1) the nondual philosophy of Advaita; (2) the Enneagram system, which describes the nine addictions and shows the way out from our compulsions and fixations to freedom; (3) the wisdom teachings of Richard Rohr and Thomas Keating (in particular), who have both written on addiction from the perspective of the Christian contemplative tradition, as well as John Main; and (4) the Hero's Journey as applied to addiction. I cite St. Ignatius of Loyola as a case study in addiction, offering some Ignatian-inspired practices and I conclude with St. Benedict's twelve-step programme for humility and a ten-step blueprint for purposeful living drawing on Platonic ethics with special emphasis on temperance as well as the (related) Eastern equivalent law of *dharma*. In the Postscript, I include some Girardian reflections, endeavouring to connect addiction with mimetic desire.

Alchemy was the mediaeval forerunner of chemistry. It was concerned with the transmutation of matter, in particular with attempts to convert base metals into gold (universal elixir). The arcane texts of alchemy symbolically portray the process of transformation: from poison to nectar – the philosopher's stone (*lapis philosophorum*). I aim to mark a similar trajectory here.

DOI: 10.4324/9781003422570-1

Chapter 1

Aspects of Addiction

Hungry Ghosts

The inhabitants of the Hungry Ghost Realm are depicted in the Buddhist literature on the subject as creatures with scrawny necks, small mouths, emaciated limbs, and large, bloated, empty bellies. This is the land of addiction. The hungry and haunted ghosts are aching for fulfilment. Perpetual emptiness characterises these creatures, as the substances and sensory objects they frantically pursue fail to satiate.

In the *Vedas* (*Garuda Purana*, verse 2.22), men who commit misdeeds become ghosts after death. These hungry ghosts are demon-like. Their story features in Buddhist, Taoist, and Hindu texts. What they have in common is that they are all afflicted with disordered desire. In Christianity, in the Book of Enoch, a certain Grigorio is depicted as endlessly yearning for a friend. This is the metaphor for inordinate or addicted desire.

The Buddhist Wheel of Life (*Bhavacakra*), which is a symbolic representation of *samsāra* (cyclic existence; the cycle of death and rebirth – reincarnation), in Tibetan Buddhism, revolves around six realms, each one of which is peopled by characters representing human existence. *Bhava* means 'being' (worldly existence, continuity, becoming) and *chakra* in Sanskrit means 'wheel' (or circle/cycle). The Wheel of Life consists of:

1 The pig, rooster, or snake in the hub of the wheel representing the three poisons of ignorance, attachment, and aversion.
2 The second layer represents *karma* (meaning 'action'), driven by intention (consequences).
3 The third layer represents the six realms of *samsāra* (see later).
4 The fourth layer represents the twelve links of dependent origination (*nidānas*). These include ignorance, choice, impressions, feelings, cravings, desire, attachment, birth, death, and rebirth.
5 The fierce figure holding the wheel represents impermanence (it is also Yama, the god of death).

DOI: 10.4324/9781003422570-2

6 The moon above the wheel represents liberation (*moksha*) from *samsāra* (*nirvana*).
7 The Buddha pointing to the circle indicates that liberation is possible. Symbolically, the three inner circles moving from the centre outward show that the three poisons of ignorance, attachment, and aversion give rise to positive and negative actions (*karma*).

The six ways of being in the world (the six realms of *samsāra*) consist of three good realms (heavenly, demi-god, and human) and three evil realms (animal [beast], ghost, hell). If the Beast Realm is driven by basic survival instincts and appetites (hunger and sexuality), in the Hell Realm, the people are trapped in states of unbearable rage and anxiety. The various realms show psychological states as much as physical domains. The Hungry Ghost Realm is populated by restless spirits with their excessive cravings and attachments. It is a frightening allegory of the addicted subject.

What Is Addiction?

Addiction is a multifaceted and multifactorial, complex issue. It is an activity whereby one engages in what is perceived to be rewarding stimuli, often short term, despite adverse consequences, which can exact a huge toll on the individual and his/her family/friends. It is any repeated behaviour (substance-related or not) in which a person feels compelled to persist regardless of its negative consequences. Addiction involves:

• Compulsive engagement with the behaviour, a preoccupation with it.
• Impaired control over the behaviour.
• Continued use of substances/addictive behaviours despite the deleterious consequences.
• Relapses despite the evidence of harm.
• Dissatisfaction, irritability, or intense craving when the object (drug/activity) is not available.

'Denial' will also usually be prevalent. The term 'addiction' derives from the Latin *addicere* and *addictus* connoting enslavement in the Middle and Late Roman Republic. In the Early Modern period, the verb 'addict' meant simply 'to attach'. The object of that attachment could be good or bad, imposed or freely chosen.

• Positive attachment
• Negative attachment

By the seventeenth century, addiction was understood in the positive sense of devoting oneself to a person or pursuit (there is no evidence for a stand-alone medical model). In the nineteenth century, addiction was seen as a medical, mental, and moral 'disease'. The two most common addictions were:

- Alcohol
- Drugs

Gambling appears to be the only behaviour satisfying both original uses – it had a strong positive connotation in its association with divination and an equally negative, stigmatising one.

Addiction attaches desire and objects of desire become obsessions. 'Attachment', which is derived from the Old French, means 'nailed to' (*attaché*). So, attachment nails down our desire for specific objects and this creates addiction. We all have addictions; addiction affects everyone. *Attachment creates addiction*. It follows, therefore, that the solution to addiction will be detachment (we will see what this might mean). All the dynamics – neurological, psychological, and spiritual – of a fully-fledged addiction are at work within each of us. The same processes responsible for addiction to alcohol and narcotics are the same for addiction to love, work, relationships, moods, etc. Addictions enslave us. The opposite of addiction, therefore, is freedom. Addictions, one might say, are the enemies of freedom.

We wonder whether addiction is 'inside us' – located intrapsychically as it were or externally in the object, whatever it may be, or our relation to substances (in-between). Addiction is a symptom of something else. We can never get enough, it would seem, of what we don't want. We don't really want the alcohol; we want what it symbolises – fullness, laughter, connection. If we can find out what we really want – our true desire – we will have the answer to addiction. Our inner *daimon* (not demon but destiny) will point us in the direction of our desire. We come into the world with a binary operation system: ego and Self. The shift I am encouraging in this book is from the former to the latter.

Psychiatry

The only behavioural addiction recognised by the two psychiatric bibles, the *DSM-5* and the *ICD-10*, is gambling. A distinction is made between, for example, drug dependence and drug addiction, with the former implying unpleasant withdrawal symptoms upon cessation. Epidemiological studies estimate that genetic factors account for 40%–60% of the risk factors for alcoholism. There are the environmental factors of lack of parental supervision, substance availability, poverty, adverse childhood experiences, emotional deprivation, behavioural problems, stressful situations and circumstances, family conflict, etc. Addiction is mainly seen as a 'biopsychosocial disorder'. The consensus seems to be that addiction is the product of genetic inheritance and environment.

Adolescence represents an unstable period in one's life, a time of greater vulnerability for developing an addiction. Aside from hormonal changes, there is peer pressure and the adolescent admixture of defiance and dependency. Studies show that those who start to drink alcohol at a younger age are more likely to become dependent later on. Those with comorbid (co-occurring) mental health disorders such as depression, PTSD, etc., are more likely to develop 'substance use disorders'. Treatments that have been put forward include therapy, twelve-step programmes, residential treatment facilities, and psychopharmacological interventions, for example, the deployment of benzodiazepines for alcohol detoxification, as well as cognitive behavioural therapy (CBT) for coping with the 'condition'. One can see how the language utilised in the debate and discourse concerning addiction is heavily influenced by an overarching physicalist and, at times, reductionist biological model. The *DSM-5* lists eleven criteria for the diagnosis of alcohol disorder:

1 Drinking alcohol in larger amounts or for longer than intended.
2 Unsuccessful attempts to cut down or stop using alcohol.
3 Spending a lot of time drinking or recovering.
4 Craving or having a strong desire to drink.
5 Failure to fulfil major obligations due to recurrent drinking.
6 Continuing to drink despite the legal, social, and family consequences.
7 Prioritising drinking over important social, occupational, or recreational activities.
8 Continuing to drink despite health warnings.
9 Continuing to drink despite it causing or exacerbating physical or psychological problems.
10 Having to drink in order to get the same effect as before (tolerance).
11 Experiencing withdrawal symptoms and taking substances as tranquilisers to relieve or avoid the symptoms (see the *Diagnostic and Statistical Manual of Mental Disorders*, 5th edition).

The CAGE (an acronym) questionnaire is a widely used assessment instrument for screening tendencies towards alcoholism. It was developed in 1968 at North Carolina Memorial Hospital and revolves around four questions:

• Have you ever tried to *C*ut down on your drinking?
• Have you ever been *A*nnoyed by people critical of your drinking?
• Have you ever felt *G*uilty about your drinking?
• Have you ever had a drink first thing in the morning (*Eye*-opener) to steady your nerves or get rid of a hangover?

Two yes responses indicate the possible presence of alcoholism.

This prevailing medical account of and approach to addiction views it primarily as a disease, which implies lesions on the brain. A central contention here is that *addiction is a disorder of attachment, not a brain disease*. I mean 'disorder' in the Platonic rather than psychiatric sense. In the latter sense, disorder refers to a functional abnormality; in the former, philosophical way of deploying the term, Plato regarded internal conflict as a paradigm case of psychic dysfunction, of inner disequilibrium – a lack of harmony or stillness in the soul, as a spiritual dis-ease.

Four Levels of Addiction

A cardinal characteristic of addiction is the gradual substitution of people by things; objects replace real people (see Gabor Maté, *In the Realm of Hungry Ghosts: Close Encounters with Addiction*; and Gerald May, *Grace and Addiction*). We can distinguish four main stages of addiction (from the National Institute on Alcohol Abuse and Alcoholism [NIAAA]):

1 Experimentation
2 Regular use
3 Risky use (misuse)
4 Dependency and addiction

The American Society of Addiction Medicine (ASAM) defines the ABCDEs of addiction thus:

- Inability to consistently *a*bstain.
- Impairment in *b*ehavioural control.
- *C*raving or increased 'hunger' for drugs or rewarding experiences.
- *D*iminished recognition of significant problems with one's behaviours and interpersonal relationships.
- A dysfunctional *e*motional response.

One frequently hears the phrase 'the addict', but the point to highlight here is that we all seek stimulation. So let us get rid of the unhelpful term 'the addict', which simply encourages us to disown our addictions, compulsions, and cravings and project or displace them onto convenient scapegoats. Pretty much everything, conceivably, can be abused or misused; the solution lies in finding measure (temperance) in all things. Dipsomania is the (pretty awful) medicolegal term for alcoholism. But objects are what they are; what matters more is the *attitude* (*bhāvanā* in Sanskrit) we cultivate towards them – our mindset, in other words, our thoughts/beliefs surrounding them. People don't have a drinking problem *per se*, they have a thinking problem.

A Tridimensional Model

What we have to do with our addictions is not flee or fight them but face them fearlessly and seek to dissolve them. This could involve psychotherapy, psychiatry, residential treatment centres, journaling, weekly meetings, various contemplative practices, Enneagram coaching, or a combination of these. There is also a plethora of groups dedicated to helping those who suffer from various addictions, including Alcoholics Anonymous, Al-Anon, SCA (Sexual Compulsions Anonymous), NA (Narcotics Anonymous), and Gamblers Anonymous. Many manuals and books have been written proposing a medical or biopsychosocial or CBT model. But we need more than medical management or cognitive containment. What is offered here is a radical, practical philosophical–spiritual approach (insisted on by the great Swiss psychologist C. G. Jung) to addiction, not as an alternative to existing templates but as an adjunct, complementary perspective. Holistic healing necessitates a tridimensional model of the human person, one which respects and gives due attention to the human being in his body (biology), mind (psychology), and heart (spirituality), to his totality/wholeness. Most treatment modalities have concentrated on the first two and largely jettisoned the last one. The addicted person will need to (re)connect with his immanent essence (Self) and seek to diminish his needy and narcissistic ego. This is the ultimate answer to addiction prescribed by the perennial philosophy and the great wisdom traditions of all time but one that has been occluded, neglected, or ignored in contemporary times. This, then, will be our primary focus.

Attachment

Part of the human condition is that we all seem to struggle with craving; such is the obsessive–compulsive nature of the ever-moving mind (*manas* in Sanskrit). The addicted person will certainly need a community (*sangha*) to support him/her. We can state two obvious truths about human beings. Their:

- Attachment to pleasure
- Aversion to pain

These are the two sides of desire. *Aversion* addictions include allergies, phobias, prejudices, and bigotries. One of the most dangerous aversion addictions is *anorexia nervosa*. Aversion addictions are mirror images of attraction addictions. (Of course, we can have strong feelings towards something which doesn't necessarily entail the presence of addiction). True addictions are habitual compulsive behaviours. It is the ego's nature to pursue pleasure and avoid pain. In Western psychoanalysis, John Bowlby made a life-study of the nature of attachment, distinguishing four types in the various volumes that comprise his *Attachment and Loss* (1997) series:

1 Secure (warm and loving bonds between a child and its parents)
2 Anxious-ambivalent (distrust of caregivers)
3 Disorganised (unmet emotional needs)
4 Avoidant (a combination of avoidant and anxious – children will display intense anger and rage and have a difficult time controlling their emotions)

Attachment is a deep, enduring emotional bond that connects one person to another. What we need as children is a secure base, a maternal containment, a holding environment. Childhood provides the template, the matrix for the subsequent maturational process. Emotional self-regulation involves creating and then extending the gap between a stimulus and a response. In the well-known 1972 Stanford marshmallow test led by psychologist Walter Mischel, a child was offered a choice between one small but immediate reward, or two small rewards if they waited for a period of time. During this time, the researcher left the room for about fifteen minutes and then returned. The reward was a marshmallow. Follow-up studies found that children who were able to wait longer for the preferred rewards tended to have better life outcomes than those who didn't. To negotiate life – its hurdles and hurts – we need to learn to calm and control our minds, to monitor and master our thoughts.

Examples of some attraction addictions: coffee, cars, gambling, gardening, golf, money, music, sleeping, soft drinks, and sports. Examples of some aversion attractions: airplanes, anchovies, death, dentists, pain, public speaking, snakes, and storms. Addictions are never good; no addiction is beneficial and some are more harmful than others. All impede human freedom. If addiction is slavery, non-attachment is freedom.

Pleasure

Sigmund Freud highlighted the importance of the pleasure principle and the reality principle in the life of a person. The addicted person will cathect his libido (attach his energy), seeking immediate reward (the pleasure principle), or he will postpone his gratification for more pleasure in the future (reality principle). A strong attachment produces a fixation. Symptoms of addictive personality (personality is addictive in its very structure) are caused *by* the addiction; they are not the cause *of* the addiction. The 'law of effect' has largely replaced Freud's pleasure principle in modern psychology. If a behaviour is associated with an effect of pleasure, then that behaviour is likely to occur more frequently (positive reinforcement). Conversely, if associated with fear or pain, it will occur less frequently (negative reinforcement). Perpetual experiences of associations between behaviour and effects (in the form of learning) are the basis of conditioning. If I do something that makes me feel good, in all likelihood, I will do it again. Attachment happens through:

- Learning (by associating a specific behaviour with pleasure)
- Habit formation (my brain makes the association between if I do this, then I will feel pleasure)
- Struggle (upon encountering any distress, my desire to do the behaviour resurfaces like a reflex)

Addiction takes place when a person ingests a substance or engages in an activity that is pleasurable to begin with but the continued use/act of which becomes compulsive and interferes with ordinary life. The pleasure, in other words, becomes painful. The addicted subject's pleasure is actually a form of *jouissance* rather than desire. *Jouissance*, according to French psychoanalyst Jacques Lacan, is beyond the pleasure principle. It's linked to the drive, to what compels the subject to transgress the prohibitions imposed on his enjoyment. The problem is this: the result of transgressing the pleasure principle is not more pleasure but pain, since there is only a certain amount of pleasure the subject can bear. Think of being tickled – there is a moment when the enjoyment becomes unbearable. *Jouissance* is the name given to this painful-pleasure principle. *Jouissance* thus involves suffering. Such 'surplus enjoyment' is perversely painful. The pain is in the too-much-pleasure. (Chemicals like morphine and amphetamines are the most addictive of all known substances.) The two properties that characterise all addictive stimuli are that they are:

1 Positively *reinforcing* (so that a person will seek repeated exposure to them)
2 Intrinsically *rewarding* (perceived as being something desirable)

There is thus immediate gratification (short-term reward), coupled with delayed damaging effects (long-term costs). Addiction, ultimately, is more about wanting (desire) than liking (pleasure).

The Spiritual Dimension

Colloquially, we hear the expression 'the demon drink' – pointing to the presence of the 'bad spirit' within (the adversary). What the alcoholic is unconsciously looking for in the bottle of spirits is spirit – the 'good spirit' within (the advocate).

Psychiatrist Gerald May asked individuals who identified as having overcome serious addiction how they succeeded. All of them described a spiritual experience (conversion) as being the one thing that put them on the path to recovery (see May, *Addiction and Grace*). This has been corroborated by the work of C. G. Jung (as we shall shortly see). So, the emphasis on the spiritual dimension has to be given priority in any attempt to help those who are addicted. 'What healed them', May writes, 'was something spiritual' (*Addiction and Grace*, p. 7).

Addictions are not limited to substances – people can be addicted to pleasing others, for example, to working, writing, etc. Addictions are compulsions outside our egoic control. Every addiction starts out as a temptation. Temptation is the first step in addiction, the original fall from grace. ('Lead us not into temptation'). In the symbolic story at the beginning of *Genesis*, the Serpent tempts Adam and Eve with the fruit of the Tree of Knowledge. Addiction invades/pervades the Garden of Eden. Addiction uses up desire, usurping it, sucking up energy. Addiction is the counterfeit of spiritual experience. One of the *Upanishads* reads: 'When all desires that cling to the heart are surrendered, then a mortal becomes an immortal'. Why? Because he becomes totally free. According to Buddhism's Four Noble Truths, suffering is caused by addiction. The Truths show a way to practice non-attachment by steering a middle course between aversion and desire.

Four Noble Truths, Three Causes of Suffering, and the Eightfold Path

First, the Four Noble Truths, which appear in many forms in the ancient Buddhist texts:

- Suffering (*dukkha*) – life is suffering (Western philosophers such as Arthur Schopenhauer and Viktor Frankl emphasised this aspect of life too).
- The origin of suffering (*samudaya*) – suffering arises with attachment/desire/craving (this has been emphasised by Christian mystics too such as Meister Eckhart and St. Ignatius of Loyola).
- The cessation of suffering (*nirodha*) – ending can be attained through renunciation of desire (*tanhä*) (this follows logically).
- The path to end it (*magga*) – the Noble Eightfold Path (unique to Buddhism, though other philosophies and religions have their equivalent).

The three causes of suffering (poisons), which we mentioned earlier, are:

- Greed (often represented as a rooster)
- Ignorance (often represented as a pig)
- Hatred (often represented as a snake)

The Eightfold Path consists of:

1 Right views
2 Right thinking
3 Right speech
4 Right action
5 Right livelihood
6 Right effort
7 Right mindfulness
8 Right meditation

Treading the Middle Path brings compassion and wisdom. For humans to be free, detachment (disidentification) from disordered desire is necessary. Detachment is not about owning nothing; it's about nothing owning us. This teaching is at the heart of all the great philosophies and spiritualities. Detachment is not so much freedom *from* desire as it is the freedom *of* desire. With freedom of desire comes the capacity to love 'disinterestedly' (without attachment). Agapeic love (as distinct from love as *eros* or *philia*) is universal. It is as non-personal as it is non-possessive. According to Taoism, the sage is detached and thus at one with all, loving the world as his own Self. The verse in the *Bhagavad Gita* proclaims poetically that the supreme 'I am' is free from attachment to all things. *Detachment is the liberation of desire.* Freedom (*moksha*) is the beyond of addiction – the Promised Land of Liberation. Just as it is not money but the *love* of money that is said to be the root of all evil, so it is that attachment (inordinate or disordered desire) to objects that is the root of all addiction. When egoic grasping, possessing, holding, hoarding, clinging, cleaving, and coveting are at play, there is attachment and most likely addiction. Desire, by definition, is never satiated but rather endlessly deferred, displaced onto other objects of desire, continually, creating a vicious circle/cycle. Addictions cripple and corrode; they compromise human freedom and dignity. Physiologically, the substance ingested alters the balance of natural body chemicals which the body must adjust to in its effort to re-establish balance (homeostasis). But by so doing, the body becomes dependent upon the external supply of the substance. May observes: 'Addiction is any compulsive, habitual behaviour that limits the freedom of human desire' (*Addiction and Grace*, p. 24).

The Five Markers of Addiction

According to May, the *five* essential characteristics of addiction are (*Addiction and Grace*, pp. 26–31):

1 Tolerance – the phenomenon of wanting or needing more of the addictive behaviour or object of attachment in order to feel satisfied.
2 Withdrawal symptoms – experienced when an addictive substance is curtailed. They are (a) a stress reaction (when the body responds with danger signals when it is deprived of something) and (b) a rebound or backlash reaction (the balance swings in the opposite reaction, for example, the withdrawal from alcohol can produce hyperactivity, while withdrawal from stimulants can result in depletion/depression).
3 Self-deception – here the 'will' fights against itself. There are mixed, murky motivations, contradictory desires, malignant mind-tricks such as denial, rationalisation, displacement, etc. that have been well described and defined by psychoanalysis.
4 Loss of willpower – intentional resolutions are hard to carry out. One fails and flounders.
5 Distortion of attention – addiction kidnaps our minds, distorting attention. Attention becomes fixed on the object of addiction, hence captured, and closed rather than open and free. One seeks the fix.

(See Damian Thompson's *The Fix: How Addiction is Invading Our Lives and Taking Over Our World*)

Addiction exists whenever one can find evidence of all five characteristics, indeed, whenever freedom is compromised. Objects of desire/attachment tyrannise and torture the addicted subject, holding him/her hostage. In denial, there is a nonrecognition of a problem even existing; in repression, there is a bottling-up and the person lives in shame and secrecy. The addicted person will procrastinate and display delaying tactics; they will also co-opt others in a web of co-dependency and deceit.

Physicians will prescribe more drugs to help people quit the primary chemicals, thus producing and proliferating multiple chemical addictions, while psychotherapists may spend months trying to ascertain a non-existent cause in early childhood. A spiritual solution is paramount. Essentially, this involves moving away from the false-self system – the ego-entity – and into our essential nature. To escape from bondage a wise man must first exercise the right discrimination between the True-Self and the Ego-self. Only then will he discover the Self as transcendental Being, Consciousness, and Bliss.

Chapter 2

Signs of Stress

There are many reasons for addiction, including familial, personal, and societal. A variety of factors can cause or at least create the conditions for addictions to become embedded in someone's life: suffering, boredom, trauma, and/or stress, to name but four. In the 1970s, research began to emerge which showed that some people who took 'addictive' substances did not become addicted, while benign behaviours, such as shopping and chocolate-eating, began to be considered as addictive (chocaholic, shopaholic). Moreover, the stress experienced by the individual taking the addictive substance or engaging in potentially addictive behaviour was now being recognised as a possible engendering factor, as having an impact on whether people became addicts or not. Addiction often appears as an attempt to deal with stress in a way that doesn't quite work for the individual. While one may gain some temporary relief from stress through the drugs or drink or behaviour one becomes addicted to, it is short-lived and can be costly emotionally, physically, and financially. One needs more and more stimulation in order to continue coping with stress. Many addictions bring further stress with them, not least in relation to the withdrawal symptoms that come when the drug in question wears off. Exposure to stress has a significant impact on addiction. A growing clinical literature indicates that there is a link between substance abuse and stress (see, for example, Nick E. Goeders's 2003 article, 'The Impact of Stress on Addiction'). Let's explore the theme of stress before returning to this subject in Chapter 9 on the Enneagram, which shows the lines of strain experienced by each personality type but also of 'security', in other words, our stress points as well as their points of release and resolution.

Defining Stress

One can take a stress test. One such test is the short ten-question Perceived Stress Scale (PSS), which is available online. Stress is wear and tear on the body, mind, and spirit, and a silent killer. Modern life bombards and besieges us with incessant impingements that can inundate and swamp us. Stress may be defined as the *feeling of being overwhelmed or unable to cope with mental or emotional pressure (strain)*. Stress increases the risk of strokes, ulcers, and heart attacks.

DOI: 10.4324/9781003422570-3

Two Types of Stress

We can distinguish between stress that is:

- External – related to the environment
- Internal – dependent on attitudes, perceptions, and beliefs

And:

- Good stress – eustress (the word was introduced by endocrinologist Hans Selye in 1976)
- Bad stress – distress

Eu means 'good' (the 'eu' in euphoria). *Dis* relates to dissonance/disagreement. A stressor is any event that causes stress in the individual. There can be:

- Overstress – hyperstress (overloaded/overworked)
- Understress – hypostress (bored/underwhelmed)

Four Categories of Stress

We can demarcate four categories of stress:

1 Crises/catastrophes (events that are completely out of our control, such as wars, earthquakes, pandemics)
2 Major life events (marriages, births, deaths that create uncertainty)
3 Daily hassles (these microstressors contribute to irritations, inconveniences, annoyances such as traffic jams, decision-making, intersubjective conflict)
4 Ambient stressors (the background environment such as noise, pollution, crowds)

The common factor of these four categories is the inconsistency between expected events ('set value') and perceived events ('actual value') that cannot be satisfactorily resolved.

Three Stages of Stress

We can further delineate three stages of stress:

1 Alarm reaction – when the stress is first presented. Here the hypothalamic–pituitary–adrenal axis and sympathetic nervous system are activated resulting in the release of hormones from the adrenal gland, such as cortisol.
2 Stage of resistance – here the body builds resistance until the body's reserves are depleted or the stressful stimulus is removed.

3 Stage of exhaustion – here the body is drained, and the person exhibits symptoms of anxiety, irritability, etc., which are part and parcel of the fight-or-flight reaction.

Four Factors in Stress Management

Stress management consists of a spectrum of techniques, tools, therapies, and coping mechanisms aimed at alleviating a person's level of chronic stress and ameliorating their subjective sense of wellbeing. Facing stress will tend to involve four factors:

- Affiliation – 'tend and befriend', dealing with stress through a social support network.
- Humour – comedic context, sharing funny stories with friends and colleagues.
- Sublimation – channelling and redirecting toxic thoughts or troubling emotions into a socially acceptable outlet.
- Reframing – cognitive reappraising or dereflecting onto more hopeful situations.

In addition to sublimation, there are other mental mechanisms through which a person has a diminished awareness of their anxiety:

- Displacement – redirecting
- Repression – removal
- Reaction formation – replacing
- Acting out – releasing

We may view defence mechanisms as an unconscious psychological operation that functions to protect a person from anxiety-producing thoughts and feelings related to internal conflicts or outer stressors. They may result in healthy or unhealthy consequences depending on the circumstances with which the mechanism is used. They are strategies that are brought into play by the unconscious to deny or distort reality in order to assuage anxiety and maintain one's self-schema. A defence mechanism becomes pathologised when its persistent use leads to maladaptive behaviour. The main purpose of them is to protect the ego from anxiety. Anna Freud's 1936 book *The Ego and the Mechanisms of Defence* is definitive. In it, she enumerates ten defence mechanisms that appear in the work of her father, Sigmund Freud.

- Repression
- Regression
- Reaction formation
- Isolation

- Undoing
- Projection
- Introjection
- Turning against one's own person
- Reversal into its opposite
- Sublimation or displacement

Anna Freud spent much of her time concentrating and researching five main mechanisms:

- Repression (the burying of a painful thought or feeling from one's unconscious)
- Regression (the falling back into an early stage of development seen as safer)
- Projection (the possessing of a feeling that is deemed as socially unacceptable but instead of facing it, that feeling is seen in the actions of other people)
- Reaction formation (the fixation in consciousness of an idea or affect that is opposite to a feared unconscious impulse)
- Sublimation (the expression of anxiety in a socially acceptable way)

The American psychiatrist George Eman Vaillant proposed a four-level distinction/classification of defence mechanisms (see his 1977 publication *Adaptation to Life*):

- Level I – pathological defences (psychotic denial, delusional projection)
- Level II – immature defences (fantasy, projection, passive aggression, acting out)
- Level III – neurotic defences (intellectualisation, reaction formation, dissociation, displacement, repression)
- Level IV – mature defences (humour, sublimation, suppression)

Resilience as the Answer to Stress

If *stress* is the reaction of a person when they feel under siege or bombarded by blows of fate, *resilience* is the attitude or ability to bounce back from adversity. *Resilience (strength of spirit) is the answer to stress. Hardiness is the antidote to hardship.* Hardiness comprises a group of attitudes and skills one needs to cultivate to build that bounce-back ability. Sociologically, the least resilient of groups – and those who are most prone to taking offence – are the 'snowflake generation', that is to say, young adults of the 2010s (those Gen Y millennials born between 1980 and 1994, and sons and daughters of the children of Baby Boomers). One rule of thumb is when things become overwhelming, remember: one task at a time, one thought at a time.

Defining Resilience

Resilience may be defined as the *positive adaptation to an adverse situation*. It's a process. The three ways we tend to approach an inauspicious event are:

1 Erupt with emotion
2 Implode with anger
3 Numb out

We need to evolve strategies to deal with stress. In *Resilience at Work*, authors Salvatore Maddi and Deborah Khoshaba state that more than four hundred studies around the world have validated hardiness as the key to resilience. They highlight three ingredients that constitute hardiness.

Three Ingredients to Hardiness

1 Commitment (involvement with people and events)
2 Control (influencing outcomes proactively)
3 Challenge (instrumental insights about how to get and grow through the stress)

These 3 C's give one the courage to face difficult or disruptive changes. Plato defined courage (one of the four cardinal virtues) as wise endurance of the soul, one that permits us to thrive and not just strive. The opposite of commitment (transformational coping) is disengaged alienation. The opposite of control (social support) is passivity and powerlessness – 'give-up-itis'. The opposite of challenge (learning) is fear and reluctant avoidance. The opposite of resilience is vulnerability.

Acute, Chronic, and Total Stress

Stress can, of course, build up. Much of it is based on the disparity between what one wants and what one gets from life. We can distinguish between:

• Acute stress
• Chronic stress

They are inversely proportionate. The less chronic stress one has, the more acute stress one can handle, and vice versa. One's total stress level is a combination of the amount and intensity of acute and chronic stress, thus:

$$Acute + Chronic \ Stress = Total \ Stress$$

Symptoms of Stress

Stressful circumstances can produce physical, mental, and behavioural symptoms.

* Physical strain: muscle tension, backaches, fatigue, stomach and intestinal upsets, influenza
* Mental strain: impatience, impaired memory, pessimism, depression
* Behavioural strain: insomnia, temper tantrums, poor performance

Intense and prolonged strain can lead to a breakdown (meltdown), wherein one succumbs to the stress. The early experiences that build resilience include childhood stress, a sense of purpose, nurtured confidence, and encouragement. The experiences that undermine resilience include, by contrast, little parental encouragement or interest, no sense of purpose, and lack of involvement. Commitment necessitates us in dedicating or devoting ourselves to a goal outside or beyond ourselves (self-transcendence). Control leads us to having and taking a hands-on approach to life (action plan). Challenge encourages us to embrace change. But what if I fall, flail, or fail? Oh, but my darling, what if you fly?

Three Sources of Feedback

What is crucial is feedback, of which there are three sources:

* Observations – the ones you make about yourself.
* Conversations – the information you receive from others.
* Effects – the impact/influence your actions have on others.

We have a *choice* about how we respond to stressful events. As the Stoic philosophers never tire of telling us: it's not the event that hurts or harms us, but the interpretation our minds give it (how we see the situation). We need to rethink things.

In every obstacle (difficulty) there lies an opportunity (solution).

Three Steps for Dealing with Stress

A three-step sequence suggests itself:

1 Broaden your perspective – try to stand back and gain a bird's-eye view of things, which the Stoics call 'the view from above'.
2 Deepen your understanding – immerse yourself in the problem-solving process or seek to understand the causes of the problem.
3 Take decisive action – seize the moment; solve the issue; devise an action plan.

It is helpful to think of the four As in terms of alleviating stress:

- Avoid (through escape)
- Alter (through communication)
- Adapt (through changing expectations)
- Accept (through making peace with)

The ABCs of Human Needs

The authors of *Resilience at Work* (Salvatore Maddi and Deborah Khoshaba) set out what they call the ABCs of human needs (and DEFs):

- Accomplishment (worthwhile/significant tasks)
- Belonging (meaningful interactions)
- Comfort (safety and security)
- Dependability (routine, regularity)
- Esteem (self-love)
- Finances (sufficient funds for a fulfilling life)

Further, one needs to come to know one's stressors, be it one's personality blockages or blind spots, communication misunderstandings, clash of wills with certain people, or external forces. And we need to develop goals – the objective will order our plans (a goal without a plan is a wish), see the big picture, and strengthen work relationships.

Six Pillars of Resilience

We can outline six pillars of resilience (see Eva Selhub, 2021):

1 Physical hardiness – fitness can facilitate resilience.
2 Emotional equilibrium – positive emotions fuel us.
3 Mental toughness/clarity – rational thinking.
4 Spiritual connection – a religious outlook minimises trauma.
5 Loving relationships – friendship and social connections.
6 Influential leadership – cultivating networks, having an impact in one's community.

From Anxiety to Excitement

We really need to change our perception of threat from negative to positive. One way of doing this is to turn anxiety (beating heart, twisted stomach, dry mouth) into excitement. This, in effect, tricks your brain because anxiety and excitement are mirror images of each other. The difference is all in the mind. So, *anxiety becomes reinterpreted by excitement*. Excitement makes the most out of the stress. To put it another way, excitement transmutes the anxiety/stress.

The ABCs of Stress

- Anxiety (too much stress)
- Boredom (too little stress)
- Challenge (to manage/monitor the stress)

The Stoic philosophers emphasise *controlling what you think, rather than changing the situation*. Stress can, of course, be controlled through our bodies (diet, sleep, and exercise), but ultimately it is to our hearts and minds that we must look for real results. Meditation is the master key to helping dissolve stress.

Causes and Cures

The work involves discovering the triggers and the solutions, thus:

- Causes (what sets me off)
- Cures (what works best)

Having a *m*eaning, a positive *a*ttitude, and *p*urpose are three core ingredients (MAP) in life, which Viktor Frankl emphasised in his logotherapy:

> If architects want to strengthen a decrepit arch, they increase the load that is laid upon it, for thereby the parts are joined more firmly together. So, if therapists wish to foster their patients' mental health, they should not be afraid to increase that load through a reorientation toward the meaning of one's life. ...
>
> Thus, it can be seen that mental health is based on a certain degree of tension, the tension between what one has already achieved and what one still ought to accomplish, or the gap between what one is and what one should become.

Viktor Frankl gives the term 'noödynamics' to this struggling and striving after a meaningful goal, which he sees as positive rather than problematic or pathological. A certain amount of tension (or stress) may be desirable if understood in this context (see, for example, Frankl, *On the Theory and Therapy of Mental Disorders*).

The Five Rs of Stress Management

Aside from logotherapy and stoicism, we can delineate five Rs of stress management:

1 Recognition of the causes
2 Relationships identified for support
3 Removal of the threat/stressor
4 Relaxation techniques
5 Re-engagement

Five Coping Skills

An alternative is the 5 Rs representing five coping skills (see Richard Blonna, 2011):

1 Rethink (how you deal with stress)
2 Relax (body and mind through pausing, mindfulness, sitting still)
3 Release (muscle tension and nervous energy)
4 Reduce (cut back on the overall volume of stressors)
5 Reorganise (increase your level of wellness across all seven dimensions)

Seven Dimensions of Wellness

Wellness is commonly viewed as:

1 Physical
2 Social
3 Spiritual
4 Emotional
5 Intellectual
6 Occupational
7 Environmental

This model (developed in the 1970s by Bill Hettler, co-founder of the National Wellness Institute) will help us to turn lemons into lemonade. We can clean and clear the lens through which we look at the world, but we can't change the picture. What this means is that we need to concentrate on what we can change/control, not on what we can't (which we seem to spend so much time stressing over). The Serenity Prayer, written by the American theologian Reinhold Niebuhr, sums up this aspect thus: 'God, grant me the serenity to accept the things I cannot change, courage to change the things I can, and wisdom to know the difference'.

A Philosophical Addendum: Snakes and Ropes

The creation itself causes no stress. It is what it is – the product of pure love, perfect and complete. It is we who find it chaotic, cruel, and capricious. There is an old story called 'The Rope and the Snake', which illustrates this point well: a man walks along a path. He sees a poisonous snake barring his way and so he turns in the opposite direction. As he returns along the same path the following morning, he finds a coiled rope on the ground. He realises that in the darkness he mistook the coiled rope as a snake, and it dawns on him that in our mental darkness (ignorance), it is difficult to see that which is. Our perception of reality can be clouded/distorted by thoughts. Ignorance can manifest itself as habit or quick judgement. When we meet our employers, we might meet our image or conception of them; in other words, we see the snake instead of the rope. So, it is possible we mistake the nature of reality. We see stress everywhere rather than ascertaining the source of the stress in ourselves. Maybe the stress we experience is the imaginary snake and the bliss of which Scripture speaks is the rope.

Perhaps what we call stress is the false use of the mind and heart. What would be a false use of the mind? Entertaining mistaken ideas about the nature of reality which we take to be true. False knowledge can contribute to a feeling of stress. In these cases, instead of meeting something or someone freshly, as it were, as if for the first time, we carry an image or thought of them from the last time, so we never really meet them as they are but as we are. In other words, we superimpose a constructed 'reality' (like a screen) on the actual reality. We conceive rather than perceive. To take another example, say you are invited to a Christmas party. Upon receiving the invite, you say to yourself, 'Oh God, it was awful last year. I didn't enjoy it. It was a long drive. Mrs X was there, and I have nothing in common with the guests' etc. A whole narrative is woven. 'I am not going to enjoy it', you say to yourself. And guess what? You don't enjoy it. In fact, you didn't go to this year's party, you went to last year's party again! In this scenario, you are thinking about the future and the future is a source of stress. This is a misuse of memory. But there is no worry in the present moment. The present moment gives you full access to your true Self. The past and the future are imaginary worlds – fictions, illusions. They are where stress appears. The cure is to awaken to the now and begin to live in the present instant. We torment ourselves with trying to change reality, endeavouring to make it conform to our minds rather than conforming our minds (and thoughts) to reality. So, we erect dichotomies between what is and what could be, between what is and how we want it to be, between what is and what should be – all according to us! We personalise everything as if we are the centre of creation. We thus resist reality. This non-acceptance causes stress. Acceptance of reality will thus eliminate stress.

Another source of stress is the belief in gain and loss. When we engage in comparisons with others, we see 'them' as having more than us or less than us and this game of 'compare and contrast' (and its concomitant, the 'blame game') merely seesaws us between frustration and short-term fulfilment. We thus need to drop all comparisons and all complaining.

A third category we can identify which contributes to a condition of stress is the belief that contentment is derived from things outside ourselves. 'If only I had a bigger house or better friends, then I would be happy'. Here we are tying happiness to an object outside our control. We have then created a dependency. This is bondage, not freedom; and it is certainly not happiness. Once dependency is created, fear enters the picture. If we put our happiness in our cabbages, Cape primroses, or cars, we will fear the loss of these. With fear comes the attempt to change that which is, which is a recipe for much misery. Cash and careers only offer temporary happiness. If possessions could make you really, truly happy, then you could make someone happy, which you can't.

Now, what might a false use of the heart look like? Here, we add feelings to facts. So, to take an example, I text a friend and he doesn't reply. I experience mild irritation which over the course of the day builds and bubbles up into annoyance then anger then fury. Before the end of the night is out, I am pacing with rage saying to myself, 'Typical. He never gets back to me. All it takes is one minute to text a response. Sure, didn't he do it two years ago too?' The following morning, I get a phone call from my friend who says, 'I am so sorry I didn't get back to you. I was taken to the hospital with stomach pains which turned out to be diverticulitis'. How do I *feel* now?! Stay with that which is – with the facts rather than adding (imaginary) feelings to the mix. Adding emotional content is yet another imposition of the ego on that which is.

Attachment is another, what I am calling, 'false use' of the mind–heart. If I attach (overidentify) with my possessions, I then become possessed by my possessions. Rather than me having them, they now have me. This is slavery as much as stress. Getting what you want and not getting it are equally problematic because there will either be an attempt to gain and retain it or there will be a fear of losing it once obtained. So, what to do with mind and heart?

We need to fill the heart with love rather than feelings, emotions, desires, and fake sentimentality. Love lightens the heart. Desires (possessions) burden the heart. If feelings are junk food for the heart, love is real food/fuel for the heart.

In terms of the mind, we need to let it fall still and fill it with reason rather than false opinion. When stillness and reason operate in the mind, then we won't mistake a snake for a rope. The two instructions/injunctions are:

- Let the mind fall still (rather than becoming distracted by many things and harbouring false knowledge).
- Let the heart be full of love (rather than fantasy and false consolation).

Then, in terms of living, we need to find true *measure*, which Plato called the virtue of temperance, a topic we will explore in Chapter 11. If we overindulge with negative thoughts or toxic emotions, we will be full of stress. In terms of health, the golden mean is not too much and not too little: right measure thus. We need to take care of what we permit to enter into our consciousness. We stand to stand guard over the gates of our minds and hearts. Perpetual vigilance (*nepsis* or watchfulness) over what we give our attention to is required. For whatever we give our attention to, grows. The present moment is *the* measure of creation. (There is a measure for everything.) To put it another way: the measure of my life is what is in front of me now (which is my teacher). Measure is minimum effort, maximum efficiency. With measure comes balance (conservation of energy) and fullness. One will then live without stress. Three practices commend themselves. Allow:

- Love to take root in the heart.
- Reason to operate in and guide the mind.
- Right measure to take place in all activity in the body.

At the centre of a storm, there is no movement, only stillness. The Self you are is still, serene, and stress-free. Like Socrates, we should desire to be relieved of opinion/ignorance, to find fulfilment in the eternal and unchanging, in the transcendent rather than the transient and temporary. Man in error chooses what contributes to his own misery/stress. Man in freedom lives in bliss.

One explanation for recent research and data showing a high concordance between stress-related disorders and addiction (especially drug addiction) is the self-medication hypothesis, which suggests that a dually diagnosed person often uses the abused substance to cope with tension associated with life stressors or to relieve symptoms of anxiety and depression resulting from a traumatic event.

The aim must be, as far as possible, to get to know our stressors/triggers and avoid or deal with them. What, though, should we do when we meet a stressful or stressed out, angry person who is polluting the atmosphere with their perturbation? First, just note that such a person is miserable, not happy, and that their stress is their slavery. Second, let their misery move you to compassion rather than criticism. The objective, surely, is to live a life of wisdom rather than worry, of what the Greek philosophers called *sophia* rather than stress.

Chapter 3

Spiritual Symbols

Ten Bulls

The Ten Ox Herding Pictures (or Ten Bulls) is a series of short poems and accompanying drawings within the Zen tradition that describe the stages of a practitioner's progress in the endeavour towards enlightenment and realising the stressless Self. The calf, bull, or ox is one of the earliest similes for meditation practice, which is recommended by Alcoholics Anonymous (A.A.). The well-known Ten Ox Herding Pictures emerged in China in the twelfth century with D. T. Suzuki. They are:

1 In Search of the Bull: 'In the pasture of the world, I endlessly push aside the tall grasses in search of the Ox. Following unnamed rivers, lost upon the interpenetrating paths of distant mountains, my strength failing, and my vitality exhausted, I cannot find the Ox'.
2 Discovery of the Footprints: 'Along the riverbank under the trees, I discover footprints. Even under the fragrant grass, I see his prints. Deep in remote mountains they are found. These traces can be no more hidden than one's nose, looking heavenward'.
3 Perceiving the Bull: 'I hear the song of the nightingale. The sun is warm, the wind is mild, willows are green along the shore – Here no Ox can hide! What artist can draw that massive head, those majestic horns?'
4 Catching the Bull: 'I seize him with a terrific struggle. His great will and power are inexhaustible. He charges to the high plateau far above the cloud-mists, Or in an impenetrable ravine he stands'.
5 Taming the Bull: 'The whip and rope are necessary, Else he might stray off down some dusty road. Being well-trained, he becomes naturally gentle. Then, unfettered, he obeys his master'.
6 Riding the Bull Home: 'Mounting the Ox, slowly I return homeward. The voice of my flute intones through the evening. Measuring with hand-beats the pulsating harmony, I direct the endless rhythm. Whoever hears this melody will join me'.

DOI: 10.4324/9781003422570-4

7 The Bull Transcended: 'Astride the Ox, I reach home. I am serene. The Ox too can rest. The dawn has come. In blissful repose, within my thatched dwelling I have abandoned the whip and ropes'.

8 Both Bull and Self Transcended: 'Whip, rope, person, and Ox – all merge in No Thing. This heaven is so vast, no message can stain it. How may a snowflake exist in a raging fire? Here are the footprints of the Ancestors'.

9 Reaching the Source: 'Too many steps have been taken returning to the root and the source. Better to have been blind and deaf from the beginning! Dwelling in one's true abode, unconcerned with and without – The river flows tranquilly on, and the flowers are red'.

10 Return to Society: 'Barefooted and naked of breast, I mingle with the people of the world. My clothes are ragged and dust-laden, and I am ever blissful. I use no magic to extend my life; Now, before me, the dead trees become alive'.

There are three types of carts discussed in Buddhism:

• Lesser vehicle – goat cart, small
• Greater vehicle – deer cart, larger
• Buddha – ox cart, limitless (the path to liberation)

The ox eats, grazes, and carries loads. The ox symbolises the moving mind, which is wayward rather than wise. 'Taming the Ox' means mastering the mind/thoughts. We need to hold the rope to the ox's nose, in other words, watch over our minds as a ranch hand watches over his cattle, keeping them from wandering off. The aim with practice is to reach the level of the white ox. This needs the discipline of the Buddha vehicle.

The Nine Stages of Tranquillity

The Ten Ox Herding Pictures depict the journey home to the true Self (Absolute). An equivalent series of stages are depicted in the Nine Stages of Tranquillity in which the mind is represented by an elephant and a monkey. These nine mental abidings within meditation, as the practice of presence to Self, are:

1 Placement of the mind – this occurs when the practitioner is able to place their attention on the object of meditation but is unable to maintain their attention for very long. Distractions and dullness of mind are among some of the hindrances.

2 Continuous placement – this occurs when the practitioner experiences moments of continuous attention on the object before becoming distracted.

3 Repeated placement – this occurs when the practitioner's attention is fixed on the object for most of the practice session and is able to immediately realise when he has lost his mental hold on the object and is able to restore that attention quickly.

4 Close placement – this occurs when the practitioner is able to maintain attention throughout the entire meditation session without losing their mental hold on the object at all; this is mindfulness. Nevertheless, this stage still contains subtle forms of excitation and dullness.

5 Taming – by this stage the practitioner achieves deep tranquillity of mind but must be watchful for subtle forms of excitation.

6 Pacifying – this is the stage during which subtle mental dullness is no longer a great difficulty, but now the practitioner is prone to subtle excitements which arrive at the periphery of meditative attention.

7 Fully pacifying – although the practitioner may still experience subtle excitement or dullness, they are rare, and the practitioner can easily recognise and pacify them.

8 Single pointing – in this stage, the practitioner can reach high levels of concentration with only slight effort and without being interrupted by any mood or movement.

9 Balanced placement – the meditator now effortlessly reaches absorbed concentration and can maintain it for hours without any single interruption.

There is also *śamatha* (literally meaning 'mind-calmness') – culmination – sometimes listed as a tenth stage.

The textual tradition of Tibetan Buddhism identifies five faults (obstacles to meditation practice) and eight antidotes within the practice of *śamatha* meditation (applied to overcome the five faults).

The Five Faults

1 Laziness
2 Forgetting the instruction
3 Laxity
4 Non-application
5 Over-application

The Eight Antidotes

(for laziness)
1 Faith
2 Aspiration
3 Exertion
4 Pliancy

(for forgetting the instruction)
5 Mindfulness

(for laxity and excitement)
6 Awareness

(for non-application)
7 Application

(for over-application)
8 Non-application

Chapter 4

Carl Jung and Alcoholics Anonymous

C. G. Jung and Bill Wilson

People take to drink and drugs (to name but two) to fill the void/existential vacuum inside. Addiction is a choice (initially) which leads (in the end) to no choice. When we reach for the computer keyboard, coffee, chocolate, cigarettes, cocaine, or credit cards – whatever the chosen method of addiction delivery – we are involved in a strategy that is not working. The aim of this strategy is to overcome our sense of separateness and its attendant experiences (loneliness, hurt, upset, anxiety, self-loathing, etc.) – our deep disconnection that drives us to addiction. The answer to this conundrum/condition is always within, never without where we tend to go looking. Far from freedom and unity, we experience only fragmentation. We are entranced and entrapped by the false-self system with its hollow promises and false beliefs, and we become prisoners of our minds, enchained in the fortress of the energetic ego. This ego-self entices, but its pleasures are shadows. Real substance emanates from the Self (our noetic or spiritual core) rather than the ego as the small or satellite self.

In withdrawing our energy and attention from objects of addiction, attachments are loosened; what we lose, over time, is the attachment itself. This is a lifelong process. The spiritual journey involves a shift of gear, from the ego or false self to the true Self (our essential nature), which is the 'real me'. The spiritual self is unaffected by anything. We become aware of the Self when we notice our own awareness, the one temporarily captured by an attachment. The presence of the Centre (Self) is unchanged and free. The ego, by contrast, creates a cage for itself. The process of this ontological shift from ego to Self is one of transformation. It is meditation rather than medication which permits us to be less bound to our addictions. Unitive or contemplative consciousness allows us to see reality just as it is. In the Christian tradition, Jesus teaches a threefold truth: (1) he insisted that we need to relinquish our attachments ('no-one can serve two masters'), (2) he preached that a life without attachment is one of liberation and love, and (3) he established a way toward fulfilment – the Good News (the Absolute as intimate immanence, in other words, the divine

DOI: 10.4324/9781003422570-5

indwelling). The Beatitudes (Sermon on the Mount) provide a testimony to freedom from attachment. Liberation comes through effort and grace ('thy will be done'). Once an addiction becomes entrenched, choice is compromised and with it, freedom.

One of the founders of Alcoholics Anonymous (A.A.) (together with Dr Bob Smith), William Wilson (Bill W), suffered from depression all his life. He had recovered from alcoholism, but not from its *root cause*, which was his attachment to pleasing others. His alcoholism was a camouflage for his attachment. This was the real issue.

Bill Wilson corresponded with C. G. Jung, the founder of analytical psychology; this was made possible by Margarita Luttichau (who was a student of Jung's and a protégé of Wilson's). Wilson had read Jung's *Modern Man in Search of a Soul* (see McCabe, *Carl Jung and Alcoholics Anonymous*). The belief began to develop that the principles of A.A. could be extended to other addictions beyond alcoholism. Wilson wrote two letters to Jung (and several to Jung's secretary, Aniela Jaffé). The first was a letter of appreciation sent to Jung a few months before the latter died in 1961. In the early 1930s, a patient of Jung's, Roland H, stopped drinking during his analysis but relapsed soon afterwards. He returned to Jung seeking help. Jung refused, telling him that nothing less than exposing himself to the experience of a genuine religious conversion (*metanoia*) could be effective. Roland H returned to the United States where he joined the Oxford Group helping many alcoholics to become sober. It was here that he underwent a spiritual awakening and stayed sober. His influence would lead, in part, to the founding of A.A. Jung replied (January 30, 1961), saying that his craving for alcohol was the equivalent of the spiritual thirst for wholeness; alcohol was a shortcut/circuit to union with God (a false spiritual experience). Wilson wrote his second letter to Jung in March 1961 asking for his views on the use of LSD for alcoholics, which Wilson favoured but Jung was antagonistic towards. Ill health prevented the now eighty-six-year-old Jung from responding; he would die on June 6 of that year. Jung felt that spirituality could not be injected by a syringe or swallowed by a pill.

Bill Wilson's experience was numinous and recounted thus: his depression was unbearable, and he cried out, 'If there be a God, let Him show Himself'. This took place in Towns Hospital. 'Suddenly the room lit up with a great white light. I was caught up into an ecstasy which there are no words to describe. It seemed to me, in my mind's eye, that I was on a mountain and that a wind not of air but of spirit was blowing. And then it burst upon me that I was a free man' (see *Alcoholics Anonymous*, p. 63). Wilson never had another drink after that spiritual awakening. Though on his deathbed in a state of delirium, he asked for three shots of whiskey. This can't be taken too seriously as he had remained sober for over thirty-six years. His was an ego collapse. The death of the ego gives birth to the Self.

Jung himself (who was nicknamed 'the barrel') at the age of fourteen visited a distillery and became 'gloriously, triumphantly drunk'. He had the experience of 'I' and 'others' merging into one. It was an experience of unity spoiled, he said, by his stupidity. He fell over drunk on the street. Later, when he was a resident medical assistant at the Berghölzli Psychiatric Hospital in Zurich where 13% of patients admitted were recorded as suffering from 'alcohol poisoning', he wrote three of these case histories. Sometime later, Jung was called to military service in the Swiss army, where he observed a high incidence of alcoholism among the young army recruits. Indeed, 13% of them were discharged, declared unfit owing to chronic alcoholism. Jung became aware of the shame surrounding alcoholism and began to understand that addiction changed one's inner world and masked psychic distress. In fact, what the addicted person was searching for was completeness, wholeness. The wholeness that comes from intoxication is an illusory wholeness to be sure, but the desire is present for numinosity (an oceanic feeling), which dissolves when one sobers up. Addiction is the search to repeat and prolong this experience of oneness. Addiction, in short (and alcoholism in particular), is the spiritual thirst for a sense of wholeness. And it is the stress on the spiritual that will become the underlying secret of enduring recovery from addiction. Only a radical conversion to something deeper and bigger and larger than the self (ego) can satisfy the soul's/psyche's yearning for meaning. This is the theme that Jung mentions in his 1961 letter of January 30 to Bill Wilson, where he ends the letter thus: 'Alcohol in Latin is "*spiritus*" and you use the same word for the highest religious experience as well as for the most depraving poison. The helpful formula therefore is: *spiritus contra spiritum*' (McCabe, *Carl Jung and Alcoholics Anonymous*, p. 136). The last line is a citation from *Psalm* 42: 1: 'As the hart panteth after the water brooks, so panteth my soul after thee, O God'. The Latin root of 'addict' connotes the idea of being a willing slave. But this is bondage not freedom. The highest form of spiritual experience (nectar of the gods) thus counters the most depraving poison, for Jung. The meaning of the Latin phrase *spiritus contra spiritum* is 'high spirit against low spirit'. High spirit counters spirits. Thus, spiritual experience is the solution to the addiction of alcoholism (and all other addictions as well, arguably).

In A.A. meetings, one can introduce oneself or 'pass'; one can say 'My name is X and I have a desire to stop drinking' or 'I am an alcoholic', but if the latter, it is important to note that this description designates only the ego in its fixation and identification, not the Self. All are welcome into the fellowship regardless of colour, class, or creed. Meetings usually last an hour; the secretary is called the 'chair' (a recovering alcoholic) and they speak for ten to thirty minutes about their experience. Members are welcomed, especially those back from a 'slip'. The preamble is read too. First names are used by way of introductions: 'My name is John, and I am an alcoholic'. Everyone says in unison 'Hi John' and at the end of the sharing 'Thank you John'. No member comments adversely on 'a share' (cross-sharing). A cup, basket, hat, or box is passed around for a collection. In Ireland and America, meetings usually end with the Lord's Prayer and the Serenity Prayer 'for those who wish to say them', after which members usually say: 'Keep coming back; it works if you work it, so work it; you're worth it'. Coffee or tea is normally served afterwards.

Themes of the Twelve Steps

According to Jungian analyst Ian McCabe, there are four main themes to the Twelve Steps of A.A. (see McCabe, *Carl Jung and Alcoholics Anonymous*, p. 59):

- Admission of powerlessness over alcohol.
- Confession of misdeeds and character defects connected with alcoholism.
- Making amends to family, friends, and colleagues.
- Having completed the exercises, then putting them into action by being of service to others, especially still-suffering alcoholics.

The process can be encapsulated thus: 'First the man takes the drink, then the drink takes a drink, then the drink takes the man'. The Higher Power/Presence is greater than the ego of the alcoholic who can do nothing without the assistance of the divine Self. An alcoholic horse thief who gives up drinking is still an alcoholic horse thief (a saying in A.A.). The purpose of the Twelve Steps is to lead to a spiritual awakening. The first step is to acknowledge that the ego is overwhelmed – this is the psychological breakthrough that permits the Self to become availed of. Spirits are a sheath imprisoning the Self.

Alchemy

Jung saw in the Great Work (*Magnum Opus*) of alchemy the psychological process of the transmutation of the *prima materia* (primal material) into the philosopher's stone (*lapis philosophorum*). According to Jung, there are four stages to the process of individuation (see Jung, *The Practice of Psychotherapy*, vol. 16):

- Confession (becoming conscious)
- Elucidation (amplification, association, creative imagination)
- Education (ego and persona)
- Transformation (assimilation)

We can similarly highlight the journey of individuation through four alchemical stages of transformation (McCabe, *Carl Jung and Alcoholics Anonymous*, pp. 70–71, cites the first three), which the addicted subject – indeed everyone called to – passes through:

- *Nigredo* (the blackening) – reaching rock bottom; the dark night of the soul; melancholia; maximum despair; chaos; disillusionment/despair; sometimes symbolised by the raven; fire; facing the shadow.

- *Albedo* (the whitening) – washing away of impurities (*ablutio*); separation or mini-death (spiritualisation); purification/purgation (catharsis); awakening; symbolised by the dove. Liberation from the shadow; emergence of soul-life; extraction of essence.
- *Citrinitas* (the yellowing) – the dawning of the solar light of one's being; the rising of the sun; the coagulation of the new personality; a 'big dream' or vision; the intuition of 'truth'.
- *Rubedo* (the reddening) – the moment of spiritual awakening, sometimes symbolised by a rose; the authentic expression of individuality.

Nigredo is the shadow which we must integrate and own (though transcend); *albedo* refers to work with one's sexual identity – the *anima* and *animus* (the contrasexual complexes); *citrinitas* is the Wise Old Man within – the inner sage or Self (here the work involves a shift of gear from the persona and ego to the Self); and *rubedo* is the philosopher's stone, the end of the Great Work, the final stage we circumnavigate to live out a new life from the centre or the Self (the archetype of wholeness). The 'will' or ego is handed over/surrendered to the care of the Self. This is the journey of individuation, of integration – the *coniunctio*. Through a process of enantiodromia, *nigredo* gives way to *albedo*, in other words, the despair which follows the descent into the unconscious becomes illumination from above. A clarity occurs and a shift in consciousness (*citrinitas*), which results in eventual and always-to-be-worked-at wholeness – the point at which a person discovers his true nature/identity. If we map the four stages of analysis with the four alchemical stages, we get the following:

- *Nigredo* – confession or catharsis. This is the shadow-work of coming to terms with our complexes; putrefaction (the burning away of the dross and excrescences of the ego).
- *Albedo* – elucidation or illumination. The development of communication between the unconscious and conscious aspects of the psyche; relationship with the Self; purification.
- *Citrinitas* – education. The focus is on forging and facilitating conscious relatedness to others and the world.
- *Rubedo* – transformation. The discovery of a personal myth and meaning through living a symbolic life; authentication (see Jung, *Psychology and Alchemy*, vol. 12).

In A.A., EGO is an acronym for Edging God Out. Over time (with patience and love), the ego will act less as master and more as servant to the Self, so that Spirit prevails over spirits. This process can be painful and is not complete with confronting (assimilating) one's personal shadow (with all its character faults), for in the best of us, there is the worst and in the worst of us, there is the best.

Ash can transform into assets. The addicted subject can move into his future without the past tripping him up in the present. (The word 'resentment' is derived from the Latin *senitire* meaning 'to feel' and *resentire* meaning to re-feel past hurts – old wounds are revisited). Just as there is no such thing as a fully individuated or integrated person, similarly there is no such thing as the recovered alcoholic. We are pilgrims on the path (*homo viator*).

McCabe concludes his book by posing a question: Are A.A. and Jungianism cults? His answer is in the negative. There are seven characteristics of a cult (see McCabe, *Carl Jung and Alcoholics Anonymous*, p. 117, quoting some researchers):

1   An unquestioning loyalty and adherence to the decisions of the leaders.
2   The presence of brainwashing techniques.
3   Proselytising others who are seen as outsiders.
4   Dependence on the group so that leaving becomes difficult.
5   Leader seen as a messiah figure on a mission to save humanity.
6   Links with family discouraged.
7   A preoccupation with money.

In sum, the key insight is *spiritus contra spiritum*, a phrase Jung is reputed to have based on a saying from William James. This wisdom, however, goes back as far as the second century when it was expounded by the Stoic emperor Marcus Aurelius as *espiritum vinci espiritus* – 'holy spirit overcomes alcoholism'.

Some Jungian Writers on Addiction

We next cite some Jungian writers on the subject of addiction. In *Drugs, Addiction, and Initiation: The Modern Search for Ritual* (1989), Luigi Zoja argues that the use of drugs in young people testifies to the resurgence of the collective, spiritual need for initiation. David Schoen, in *The War of the Gods in Addiction: C. G. Jung, Alcoholics Anonymous and Archetypal Evil* (2009), asserts that addiction is a malevolent force not amenable to medication or reason or analysis but that the Twelve Steps work precisely because it's a spiritual approach adapted to one's shadow side. Sam Naifeh similarly maintains in his article 'Archetypal Foundations of Addiction and Recovery' (1995) that the loss of containment is the hallmark of addiction. Underlying the Twelve Steps is the archetype of initiation in the form of containment, confrontation with the shadow, and the relinquishing of egoic control in favour of the Self as the organising principle of the psyche. Joseph Redfearn locates the addict part of the personality in our various subpersonalities as set out by him in his *My Self, My Many Selves* (1994).

Finally, we may note Jung's letter to Dominican theologian Victor White, OP (1902–1960) concerning mescaline, a naturally occurring psychedelic known for its hallucinogenic effects comparable to those of LSD and psilocybin:

Is the LSD drug you're referring to mescaline? It has indeed very curious effects, of which I know far too little. I don't know either what it's psycho-therapeutic value with neurotic or psychotic patients is. I only know there is no point in wishing to know more of the collective unconscious than one gets through dreams and intuition. The more you know of it, the greater and heavier becomes your moral burden, because the unconscious contents transform themselves into your individual tasks and duties as soon as they become conscious. Do you want to increase loneliness and misunderstand-ing? Do you want to find more and more complications and increasing re-sponsibilities? You get enough of it.

If I once could say that I had done everything I know I had to do, then perhaps I should realise a legitimate need to take mescaline. If I should take it now, I would not be at all sure that I had not taken it out of idle curiosity. I should hate the thought that I had touched on the sphere where the paint is made that colours the world, where the light is created that makes shine the splendour of the dawn, the lines and shapes of all form, the sound that fills the orbit, the thought that illuminates the darkness of the void.

There are some impoverished creatures perhaps, for whom mescaline would be a heaven-sent gift without a counter poison, but I am profoundly mistrustful of the pure "gifts of the gods", you pay very dearly for them.

This is not the point at all, to know of or about the unconscious, nor does the story end here. On the contrary, it is how and where you begin the real quest. If you are too unconscious, it is a great relief to know a bit of the collective unconscious. But it soon becomes dangerous to know more, be-cause one does not learn at the same time how to balance it through a con-scious equivalent. That is the mistake Aldous Huxley makes, he does not know that he is in the role of *Zauberlehrling*, sorcerer's apprentice, who learned from his master how to call the ghosts but did not know how to get rid of them again.

(Jung, *Letters*, vol. 2, 1951–1961, p. 172)

Chapter 5

The Philosophy of Advaita

The Spiritual Self

The Self cannot be addicted to anything as it doesn't attach to anything. Humanity's ultimate sickness is threefold:

• Ignorance
• Stupidity
• Insanity

These problems are *mental* ones. The ultimate medicine is nondual understanding (*advaita* meaning 'not two'). About 99.9% of people are addicted to something, but this something is not the object of attraction/addiction at all. It's merely a vehicle used for escaping or trying to cope. It's ultimately about what we are thinking *of*, not what we are addicted *to*. It all starts with cognition, with thinking–feeling–behaving. Habitual, mechanical thinking triggers the desire of humanity in a twofold manner:

1 A primary desire for control
2 A secondary desire for power (in order to be able to control)

It's a certain way of ego thinking that leads to attachment, which is the core/cause of addiction. So, the solution will involve a certain amount of unlearning. It will consist of transitioning from the false-self system (ego) to the authentic Self, as I've said. We use substances or people like transitional objects (in Donald Winnicott's sense), for example, a child will use a comfort blanket or soother to assuage his anxiety. At the age of six, it's understandable. Children desire to control their environment and because they can't, they try to avoid uncomfortable situations by using transitional objects. As adults, these objects usually fall away. The addicted subject, however, maintains them. All psychological problems are rooted in the personality.

DOI: 10.4324/9781003422570-6

A Desert and a Garden

We can distinguish between a desert and a garden. The desert (where a number of prophets fought their inner demons – think of Moses, Elijah, Buddha, John the Baptist, the Desert Fathers, Muhammad) depicts humanity's struggle with addiction; it's a place/state of trials, toxic thoughts, temptations, tribulations, and tricks. Jesus was faced with a triple test of temptation – all consequences of attachment. The garden (such as the Edenic paradise) is a place/state of flourishing. Gardening of the desert takes work. *Freedom from attachment is liberated love.* We hear the phrase 'reformed' character. Reformation consists of substituting destructive actions for constructive ones. Dereflection, where we put our minds on more meaningful activities and pursuits, is deliverance from toxic dependency. This path/process requires honesty (acceptance and acknowledgement), humility (self-awareness), responsibility (not its refusal through the mechanisms of displacement or denial), community (support), and simplicity (one day at a time, one foot in front of the other, step by step – patience and perseverance, so). KISS: Keep It Simple, Stupid (simple but no simpler). Another acronym might help with maintaining progress – keep it SMART: Specific, Measurable, Attainable, Realistic, and Time-bound.

There are little addictions (harmless) and large addictions (harmful). The Desert Fathers were the first to practice prayer and Christian meditation in the deserts of their hearts. These contemplative men and women of the third and fourth centuries lived lives of solitude in the caves and wild places of Egypt and Syria. In practising the prayer of the heart, they became wise and compassionate depth psychologists. They identified what forms our distractions (aversions and desires) assumed, calling them 'afflictions' rather than addictions. *All addictions are behaviours based on mistaken beliefs.* Their suggestions and solutions were simple: instead of fighting with our inner demons, locked in chronic combat, we can choose to starve them of attention and put our minds on the mantra/sacred word in the gentle daily discipline of meditation. We can't vanquish the ego with violence; what we can do is change the direction of attention. We transcend the ego by ignoring it. Over time, a modicum and measure of sobriety and stability returns, and we become anchored once more in the Self. 'Meditation' derives from the Latin *in medio stare*, which means 'to rest in the centre'. If silence enables us to let go of thoughts, stillness helps us let go of desire.

When one says or sounds the mantra/sacred word, one is not attending to the ego. Healing begins. Meditation is *the* way of following the eleventh of the Twelve Steps, as we seek 'through prayer and meditation to improve our conscious contact with God as we understand Him, praying only for knowledge of his will and the power to carry that out'. Meditation may, of course, have to be augmented by clinical support, group work, detoxification, therapy, etc. in any recovery programme. But meditation or prayer is the fulcrum, the part which holds together the rest. Like the Desert Fathers, we should seek a state of *apatheia*, which is not the same as *acedia*. If the former is the absence of attachment, the latter is the absence of care (lethargy, lack of interest and initiative). The aim is to secure salvation/redemption. 'Salvation' in Latin, Greek, and Hebrew refers to 'safety'. This is what is at stake – our safety and sanity.

Ignorance as the Cause of Addiction

Addictions, according to the Indian philosophy of Advaita, are due to ignorance, to not knowing the true nature of the way things are (to our mistaken beliefs, as we called them earlier). The individual feels separate and isolated – hence his dissatisfaction and discontent. The desire for lasting happiness and the desire to overcome separateness leads to addiction. But the addictive substance, as Freud noted in *Civilization and Its Discontents*, only gives momentary relief. It may numb/nullify feelings of despair, of grief or guilt, but long term it is not effective. All forms of addiction may be seen as an attempt to get rid of the feeling of separateness and isolation. Alcohol, drugs, and smoking all have their origins in the gross body, in the feeling of being limited and located. When we see we are not separate, the seeking/searching ends. Fear and desire are the two faces of the apparent separate self – they are the two most common forms of resistance to that which is. We thus have:

- The apparent separate self.
- Resistance to what is.
- The search for happiness via certain substances/objects.

In a sense, these three are synonymous. They are really one. They can be subsumed under the term 'ignorance' (the lack of true knowledge concerning that which is). Reality, according to Advaita Vedanta, is nondual. The resistance to and rejection of that which is is the primary cause of addiction. It has its origin in the belief that what we are (which is awareness) is limited to and located in a physical body. To be sure, we are embodied beings, but the Self is not the body. The body ages, grows, and dies but the I is eternal. This identification with the physical form of the body brings much misery. It creates an apparent entity: the ego. When this happens, the real I – awareness – becomes the limited I of the imaginary, separate, isolated body entity. This body is subject to changes and moods and endless becomings, and because it is always threatened with the possibility of non-existence, fear begins to foster and form in the heart, together with its natural corollary, desire. The greatest fear becomes the fear that 'I' will be no more, that 'I' will disappear or die. The desire then is created which yearns to substantiate this fleeting entity that we believe we are in order to perpetuate/prolong its apparent existence. This fear and desire manifest in many ways, not least in the endless inner chattering of the mind, in its constant commentary. This repetitive background noise takes us away from that which is. In a way, daydreaming, fantasy, muttering, complaining, moaning, resisting, or idle speech, is the primal addiction. It is captured attention. 'What is' is experienced as tedious, threatening, torrid, or terrible, so we construct a dreamworld which we fill with mechanical thoughts as a diversion, distraction, an escape from discomfort. Most of our thinking and endless worrying and imagining serve no purpose at all, especially ruminating on the past or anticipating the future. The problem is, over time, such thinking no longer serves to assuage our anxiety or overcome our dis-ease – our feelings of separateness. We begin to turn to stronger forms of avoidance, to substances which block out the perceived pain. We overeat or overwork; we manically pursue money or position or status; we smoke and drink to excess, unable to find measure (temperance) in our indulgences. We deny the truth of things (what is, i.e., the true nature of reality) and the now (present moment). Society condemns some of our addictive choices and condones others. Behind all addiction is thinking at the level of the mind and feeling at the level of the body. Identifying the 'I' (who we are in truth) with the physical body is the root of all suffering, which addictions seek to alleviate but in a mistaken manner. And the hysterical hunt for happiness, which is its counterpart, is just another subtle form of contemporary addiction.

What, then to do? We need to go to the root of the matter, to the source of the apparently separate self; we need to awaken and see clearly so that we can become free of illusion, mistakes, deception (*maya*), and fear. Addiction is merely a symptom of a much deeper malaise – that of the separate ego, the veiling of awareness. We need to explore this at the level of the mind (through self-enquiry or dialectic, which we are doing here) and come to see that there is no evidence for the belief in the separate I, and at the level of the feelings/emotions, those passions of the soul, as well (primarily done through some form of contemplative practice).

One rule of thumb: if, for example, a person is addicted to pornography and they are feeling the impulse to watch some, simply pause. Put a space between the stimulus and the response. Then extend it. This requires ongoing patient practice. At first, the space between won't be peaceful, but *padam, padam* – one step at a time. Also, be attentive to your thoughts: What are they telling you? What story have you fabricated, constructed, superimposed on that which is?

See a feeling for what it is – a raw bodily sensation, neutral or negative. But we don't have to feed our fantasies and feelings; we can deprive them of oxygen by not giving them attention. Their job is to keep moving. By not engaging with them, we move them on. Once the mechanism of the separate self has been seen through (understood and felt), old patterns of behaviour and belief diminish and dissipate. This process will take time, as addictions are powerful. We just permit the panoply of thoughts and feelings to arise without commentary, attachment, or judgement in the mind or heart. We simply observe them, witness them, and wish them well on their way. Their ferocity will die down in due course. It is this open, allowing, indifferent, detached presence which restores the 'I' to its rightful place as pure presence, the seat of the witness Self.

If psychiatry and psychotherapy offer containment, Advaita offers a cure. There is no sadness or stress, no anger or agitation in the serene Self. From such a clearing (enlightened state), we can see addiction for what it really is: idolatry. Why? Because every addiction seeks to absolutise that which is only relative. If addiction gives up everything for one thing – the toxic substance (for example) – what is called recovery is the giving up of that one thing for everything else.

The Natural Desire for Happiness

Our essential nature does not share the limitations of our body–mind. The question becomes, what exactly is a reliable source of lasting happiness and peace, given that everything is changing all the time? We naturally desire happiness, as philosophers from Aristotle through Aquinas to contemporary thinkers haven't tired of telling us through the aeons. Three existential questions arise:

- What is a sustainable source of happiness?
- What is the nature of reality (and our relationship to it)?
- How should we live?

The first thing to state is happiness is our birthright; it belongs to the nature of being itself. So, why don't I always experience happiness? Happiness is veiled but can be availed of. We aren't happy because we don't know the Self. We have become ensnared and enslaved by the ego-entity. We live in a trance. Advaita provides us with knowledge of our essential Self, not just the body–mind conglomerate/amalgam. What is the Self? It is that which remains with us all the time. It is not a thought, not a feeling, not an activity (*neti, neti*) – these come and go. The Self endures. The I that is always there is the Self. It's who I am in truth – pure being. It's like the screen before the movie. The screen remains constant through the comings and goings in the movie we're watching. The screen is akin to awareness; the movie is all our experiences. The screen is the Self – the knower of the known (all our thoughts, feelings, perceptions, sensations), the witness, awareness, presence, observer. The Self reveals itself as consciousness when I step back from the contents of consciousness. The 'I awareness' is aware of body, mind, and world. It is prior to any identification and activity. By contrast, the ego proclaims: 'I am tired' or 'I am thirty' or 'I am thirsty'. I am aware of all these states, so I am not these states. *I* am not tired or thirsty or thirty. We don't have to change our thoughts or feelings (the actions in the movie, as in cognitive behavioural therapy, for example). We simply watch them like a movie.

The 'I' is not an addict; only the ego-entity is addicted. The whole human race is addicted to thinking. Such thinking is cheap, legal, and harmless, but it is also fallacious. Thoughts are like trains and the mind is like a train station, but we don't have to keep jumping onto each train that pulls up. If I am aware of being fed up or full, fickle, frustrated, fascinated, or fixated, then who is the 'I' that is aware? Thoughts and feelings and identifications and attachments and addictions hold us hostage. The movie mesmerises us. Every time we take a step back to the seat (in the movie theatre or cinema) of awareness or go 'backstage', it gets easier – the power of experience weakens. We become established, anchored in awareness (our new and stable Centre). The Self is our true nature; we mistakenly think it's our experience – me talking or troubled or thinking. But it is obvious that I am not always those things. If the ego (*Aham-kara*) is 'I am such and such', the Self is simply 'I Am' (*Aham*) – an unqualified being, limitless, infinite, and free, of which there is only one, not two or ten thousand or nine billion. In Advaita, we subtract, we don't add; we return to simplicity, unity. All existence derives from the 'one without a second' (*ad--vaita*). The real world is infinite not an isolated or independent being. I am the one that is aware; I am *that* (*tat tvam asi*) that's aware, and awareness is not conditioned by experience. The Self is supreme awareness. Everyone is your Self (isn't this what 'love your neighbour as yourself' must mean?). If in a play, I act the part of Hamlet, there is still just the one person playing, not two people – *one* consciousness as the source of all. Only the *ahankara* is an alcoholic or a gambler. The Self is unattached, non-addicted. The Self is the 'higher power' of which Alcoholics Anonymous speaks. It is far greater than the meagre and mediocre and mean personality. When we identify with the small self, we feel incomplete and inadequate and so we cling and cleave and seek to acquire. We identify with the contents/objects of our experiences or addictions. This is the source of so much sorrow, suffering, and stupidity.

We are aware of our thoughts, feelings, perceptions, and sensations, but we tend not to be aware that we are aware. We don't ask what it is that is aware of this flow of thoughts, feelings, etc. The knowing of our being (or, rather, awareness's knowing of its own being in us) is our primary experience. It's the experience of 'I am' or 'I am awareness'. The Self is awareness – constant, unintermittent. The object of Self-enquiry or *atma-vichara* (the work of Ramana Maharshi, for example) is to find the true nature of the Self as Awareness, of I-am-ness. By paying close attention to the 'I'-thought, this 'I'-thought will disappear and only 'I-I' or Self-awareness remains (Self-realisation/liberation).

I have a body, but I am not my body. I have emotions, but I am not my emotions. I have intellect, but I am not my intellect. My thoughts, bodily sensations, and feelings come and go. I merely observe them. So, I am not identical to the *contents* of my consciousness. What, so, am I? I am pure *consciousness* – complete, perfect, whole. (For further discussion of Advaita, see my trilogy *The Nine Faces of Fear*; *Between Speech and Silence*; and *Dynamics of Discernment*.)

Addictions and Energy

According to ancient wisdom – the Indian philosophies of Advaita and Ayurveda – there are three qualities permeating and pervading all of creation. They are called *gunah*. All objects, thoughts, actions, and relationships have one or the other of these three qualities, or a combination of two or all three, but one will always predominate. They are always present and always in competition with each other. In Sanskrit, they are known by the names of *sattva*, *rajas*, and *tamas*. *Sattvic* means simple, sincere, honest, undiluted, lucid, luminous, spiritual. *Rajasic* means regal, glamorous, glittering, seductive, splendid, strong, exciting. *Tamasic* means dulling, dictatorial, sinister, fearful, harmful. Kindness would be sattvic, anger rajasic, and revenge tamasic. Thus:

* *Sattva* – serene and shining
* *Rajas* – stimulating and strenuous
* *Tamas* – slothful and sluggish

Sattvic is buoyant and boundless, elegant, and simple. Rajasic is moving and active, extravagant, and excessive. Tamasic is heavy and dominating, dark, and depressing. When these principles are in balance, our lives express themselves in physical, emotional, and spiritual wellbeing. If *sattva* is steadfast, *rajas* is scintillating, while *tamas* stagnates. If *sattva* seeks happiness, *rajas* seeks success, and *tamas* wants control. Too much *rajas* leads to the conditions of *tamas*. In meditation, these two forces dissipate, and pockets of *sattva* proliferate instead. We want to be aiming at a sattvic lifestyle. In life, we need to develop the right measure and mix of sattvic, rajasic, and tamasic. But at the secret centre of our being, there are no compartments or categories. Pausing during the day and meditation bring order to the being and the interplay of the three *gunah*. There are some parallels with Plato, who viewed the human being as consisting of three layers: appetitive, spirited, rational. Of course, this is a virtual not real distinction (the soul is indivisible and immaterial). We can put it this way:

Heart	Reason	Sattva
Head	Courage	Rajas
Gut	Temperance	Tamas

Tamas is the desiring element in the soul/psyche. It aims at the satisfaction of the senses; its highest end is pleasure, and its constant characteristic is ignorance. *Rajas* denotes emotional energy and the impulse to succeed in the world. At its best, it possesses the virtue of temperance. *Tamas* is restless, just like the addicted subject. *Tamas* attaches. Its ends are power and profit. *Rajas* stands midway between *tamas*, which can know nothing, and *sattva*, which is capable of understanding everything. At its best, it possesses the virtue of courage. *Sattva* denotes the higher faculty of intelligence but also the quality of goodness and stability. It will guide us aright; on it depends all the virtues but one in particular: practical wisdom (*prudentia*). The summit of its attainment is the right performance of all duty (*dharma*). These three qualities run through the whole of the created existence/phenomenal world. *Tamas*, being the lowest quality, is bad; *sattva* being the highest, is always good; while *rajas* being the intermediate quality is partly bad and partly good. We might simply describe them as:

- Desire – appetite; related to inertia and illusion. It can never lead beyond a ceaseless recurrence of wants and satisfactions. This has an obvious affinity with addiction.
- Emotion – attaches through bonds of affection. It leads us to some sort of attainment and achievement.
- Intelligence – this state is one of balance and produces harmony/equilibrium, which is very different from restless struggle and striving.

The Goldilocks principle is apposite here: the analogy is from the children's story, *The Three Bears*, in which a young girl named Goldilocks tastes three different bowls of porridge and finds she prefers porridge that is neither too hot nor too cold, but one which has just the right temperature. This 'just the right amount' is *measure*, the Middle Way, the *metaxy*. It is what the addicted subject (all of us) must find on the path to sobriety and sanity.

The greatest number of people in society belong to the tamasic group, a smaller number to the rajasic group, and very few indeed to the sattvic group. The three parts of the soul correspond to three classes in society, for Plato:

- Traders: Tamasic
- Warriors and administrators: Rajasic
- Priest-rulers, philosopher-kings, educators: Sattvic

Tamas is needed to gain the satisfaction of our desires. *Rajas* provides the stimulus needed to excel, succeed, and manage/administer. It is needed to safeguard our social wellbeing and consolidate our affections (friendships). *Sattva* supplies the motive and means to be just and good (virtuous). The crown of its excellence is known as *dharma* (which is more than duty – it denotes the very function or purpose of something). *Dharma* is the complete stage of the development of anything – its evolution, fruition, the law of its own being, its fulfilment. For example, the *dharma* of a plant is to produce flowers and fruit. The *dharma* of fire is to burn and give heat. The *dharma* of the soul is to have all three *gunah* working perfectly together in proper measure. (*Dharma* literally means 'that which holds the soul to God'. Plato's equivalent term is *Dikaiosune* – 'righteousness'/justice.) *Dharma* is the meaning of our life, its *raison d'être*, its inner *Ikigai*, and this is what the addicted subject was searching for (unconsciously) all along. *Dharma* means doing the right thing rightly for us; it is the eternal law of life. Seen in this light, *sattva* is right desire. It is this quality that we are much in need of. The 'addict' is embedded in tamasic desire – here the aim of desire is to repeat the same satisfaction constantly, again and again and again. The character of these tamasic desires is the recurrence or repetition of sameness, of want and of satisfaction. Addiction is a hamster-wheel existence. Once the desire is attained, it is followed by a desire for new objects. It never stops, until death. Tamasic desires move in a stationary, vicious circle of stagnation. Rajasic desires, for their part, endlessly rush on from one object to another. (*Rajas* is nearer to *sattva* than is *tamas*.)

Some Examples

There are three kinds of food: sattvic foods, which are soft and sweet, producing health and vitality; rajasic foods, which are sour and pungent, spicy, and salty, producing disease and pain; tamasic foods, which are tasteless, produce lethargy and dullness, and are difficult to digest. Alcohol and drugs fall into the tamasic category – tamasic food will lead to tamasic behaviour (the same is true for all the *gunah*, each in their own way). There are three kinds of service: sattvic service, which expects no reward in return; rajasic service, which is offered for gain and reward; and tamasic service, which may be offered in faith but in which there is no fervour. There are three kinds of understanding: sattvic, which creates synthesis and sees unity and wholeness; rajasic, which causes disunity and separation; and tamasic, which focuses on the part and sees it as if it were whole. There are three kinds of action: action performed without attachment and desire is sattvic; action performed under stress for gratification is rajasic; and action performed in ignorance without regard for consequences is tamasic. There are three kinds of person: a person with no ego who is unperturbed by both success and failure is sattvic; one who is swayed by passion and greed is rajasic; while the person who is deceitful and dependent is tamasic. There are three kinds of communication: the sattvic way dialogues and seeks to understand; there is no dogma or desire to convert or critique. The rajasic way bargains and bribes and seeks to convince. The tamasic way is the way of monologue; it cajoles, imposes, and threatens. In terms of buildings/ dwellings, there are homes (sattvic) that are pleasing and serene. There are rajasic buildings – palaces and pyramids, castles, and cathedrals. Tamasic buildings are functional and useful – bunkers and barracks, schools, and shopping malls are examples. Tamasic structures are built with cement and concrete, plastic, and steel.

Living in the present moment is sattvic; dwelling on the future – planning and projecting – is rajasic; while living in the past is tamasic, deflecting our attention from living in the here and now. Ultimately, the three *gunah* relate to our state of mind. Sattvic leaders use their power for the good; rajasic rulers influence through authoritarianism and control. It's important to try to eliminate tamasic tendencies in our lives and try to reach sattvic solutions – these move slowly but surely.

- *Sattva*: preservation – calmness, clarity, creativity.
- *Rajas*: reaction – changing and active energy.
- *Tamas*: distraction – inertia and passivity.

The steady flow of a stream is sattvic. A waterfall is rajasic. And when the water is blocked or becomes polluted, that state is tamasic. The sattvic state is as simple as it is sublime; it is spiritual, subtle, and self-organising. *Sattva* is about being rather than having or doing. It values stillness and silence, is appreciative, aware, and affirmative, and seeks wholeness and harmony. Sattvic energy leads to freedom. By comparison, a rajasic person wanders from one shiny object to another in a supermarket of desire, seeking pleasure and endless, shallow stimulation, resorting to drugs in his/her search for nirvana. If *sattva* is a state of effortless, natural being, *rajas* is the state of active seeking and constant longing. The rajasic way of life celebrates speed and success and admires the powerful and the prestigious. *Rajas* relishes money and hungers after comfort and convenience. The tamasic tendency is toward darkness; it is fearful and secretive and associated with clubs and casinos (gambling) and the underworld.

Indian philosopher Vinoba Bhave, the spiritual successor of Mahatma Gandhi, employed the metaphor of a lantern to understand the three *gunah*:

> A lantern has a glass exterior which gets filled with black soot inside, and the light is dimmed; that dark soot is tamasic. Dust also falls on the lantern, which further diminishes the light; this is rajasic. With attention and mindfulness, the black soot and the grey dust are removed, and one is able to receive the full benefit of the light through the transparent glass; the clean glass is sattvic. Our aim in life should be to develop such a clarity and purity that the clear light of truth can shine through.
>
> (as cited by Satish Kumar in *Spiritual Compass*, p. 141)

The three *gunah* are a compass for life. Once we live our true nature, we are on a sattvic path. However, when we deviate, we fall into the rajasic and tamasic trap. Materialism could be described as rajasic existence. Land, labour, and literature are all commodities to be consumed. The true nature of the soul is sattvic. Leading a sattvic life is the real solution to the bipolarity/seesaw swinging of *rajas* and *tamas*, and thus of addiction.

Cocaine gives an initial rajasic rush of euphoria, boundless energy, and boosted self-confidence. Its tamasic consequences, however, include insomnia, headaches, tremors, and paranoia. Crack (base/rocks/crystal) has similar effects to cocaine, just more extreme. It gives mental exhilaration, but the crash afterwards leads to drowsiness and depression. Methamphetamines likewise give a sense of a euphoric rush but crash after, leaving symptoms of aggression and violence in their wake. Ecstasy (pills/MDMA) provides extreme energy, artificial empathy, and an enlarged sense of pleasure. The inevitable crash comes with tiredness, lack of motivation, nausea, and sometimes seizures. Mephedrone is like 'e'. We hear the terms 'uppers' and 'downers', which characterise the bipolarity of drugs as they oscillate between mania and melancholia. Depressants are tranquilising drugs that delay certain brain functions; they block pain and alter mood. Heroin (smack/gear), for example, binds to opioid receptors in the brain resulting in a 'heroin high', but the crash results in weak limbs and drowsiness. Stimulants, by contrast, help the person stay awake and alert. Cannabis (marijuana/grass/dope/pot/weed) provides vivid sensations and produces laughter as well as paranoia. Amphetamines, such as speed, increase sociality and activity. This is by no means an exhaustive list, just some examples of the effects of the drugs on the somatic system. So, we can see that some substances produce initial *rajas* (alcohol and cocaine, for example) but ultimately end in a tamasic state. The artificial, seemingly sattvic state that some drugs provide will always wear off. We can, therefore, state that, *all addictions are tamasic*. More *sattva* is/should always be the response to the play of *rajas* and *tamas* within the human being.

Sattvic Spirituality

Religion is made up of three rajasic dimensions and one sattvic. The *institutional* dimension consists of rules, of pomp and power, and is run on rajasic patterns. The *aesthetic* dimension relates to forms of music, poetry and paintings, architecture, and ceremonials. The *ethical* dimension (loving your neighbour, selfless service) preaches freedom from ego. The *mystical* dimension (Sufism for Muslims; the Kabbalah in Judaism; and Christianity has the teachings of Meister Eckhart, Julian of Norwich, etc.) emphasises the divine indwelling – the immanent Absolute. The sattvic mystical experience is rooted in a sense of the sacred (see Kumar, *Spiritual Compass*, p. 51). The three sattvic virtues par excellence, according to Kumar, are trust, participation, and gratitude. Trust is the antidote to fear; tamasic fear and insecurity are at the root of addictions. Participation is the answer to isolation, and the attempt to relinquish personal control and manipulation of the miracle that life is. Slowness and simplicity are sattvic qualities. Capitalism is the economics of addiction. The spiritual life is more about subtraction/surrender rather than addition. By contrast, addiction is always about *addition* in the frenetic pursuit of what turns out to be illusory shadows of happiness. Gratitude, for its part, stops us from complaining and criticising. In the sattvic worldview, there is no separation between matter and spirit, the natural and the supernatural (see Kumar, *Spiritual Compass*, pp. 57–62). This is a sketch as to how we can proceed, addiction-less but nonetheless filled up with *sattva* rather than substances. For *sattva* is the real solvent.

All our tossing, turning, and thinking can be halted by pausing between two activities (even for a nanosecond) and the daily discipline of meditation or prayer. which enables addicted humanity to move from *tamas* to transformation and from 'me' (the illusion and ignorance of thinking I am an isolated and separate individual) to 'we' (monanthropism/universal humanity), for the entire universe is encapsulated in me. Ownership is rajasic; stewardship is sattvic. We are trustees and guardians of the earth. This insight, based on non-dual unity, puts us in league not at loggerheads with nature, as we take the step from desire to delight and from compulsion to contemplation.

'Be the change you want to see in the world', was Gandhi's pragmatic and prophetic proclamation. Change occurs from the groundswell and grassroots; it's bottom-up. Kumar proposes an eleven-point programme for sattvic (non-addicted) action (see Kumar, *Spiritual Compass*, pp. 86–89).

1 Change our attitudes (alter our mindset from reacting to recognising and respecting life's beauty; ceasing seeing the earth as a place to plunder and pillage)
2 Live simply (eco-friendly)
3 Consume less (live more lightly; there is enough in the world for everyone's need but not for everyone's greed, as Gandhi put it)
4 Waste not (a tamasic sin; instead reuse and recycle)
5 Use no harmful products (organic ones if possible)
6 Walk (come into contact with nature)
7 Bake bread (rather than pumping ourselves with processed food)
8 Meditate (for replenishment; devote at least half an hour in the day to solitude, stillness, and silence)
9 Work less (keep track of the work-life balance lest exhaustion sets in)
10 Be informed (study; stay curious)
11 Organise (be awake and alert and speak out against exploitation and injustice; speak truth to power)

In such a sattvic (and holistic) scheme, ethics, economics, and ecology all interlink: ethics is justice at the individual level, philosophical economics is justice at the societal level, while systems' ecology ensures justice at the planetary level. Everyone, but especially addicted subjects, needs a vision laden with values. Gandhi's was one such. His trinity consisted of:

- *Sarvodaya* – 'the upliftment of all' (peace and prosperity for everybody, not just a few, as is the case in both capitalism and socialism; more biocracy than democracy, as the former encompasses all life including animals and the earth)
- *Swaraj* – 'self-government' (small-scale, social transformation – decentralised and self-directed)
- *Swadeshi* – 'local economy' (production by the masses rather than mass production)

Souls suffer because of attachment and desire. Living within limits (from a position of need rather than greed, and measure rather than pleasure) is to move from the anguished cry of the addicted person's 'more, more' to 'enough now': from *tamas* to temperance. Truth ultimately means understanding the real, nondual nature of reality itself. *Sattva* is the original, natural high.

Chapter 6

The Twelve Steps of Recovery

Many alcoholics and those addicted to other substances have turned to various twelve-step programmes as a blueprint for living. The steps are compatible with all world philosophies and spiritualities, especially Advaita, and are pertinent to those who may not self-identify as 'addicts' but who live an addictive existence. The emphasis throughout the steps is to realise that real power comes from something greater than one's egoic self. For the addicted subject, more is never enough. Though the Twelve Steps of the Alcoholics Anonymous (A.A.) programme are alcohol specific in language, they are not alcohol specific in application. It is important to note the historical context: they were written by Christians and the language of the 'Big Book' reflects a time, a place, and a particular religion. Nonetheless, the message and specific steps have universal significance.

The Twelve Steps

Step One

> We admitted we were powerless over alcohol [substitute here and throughout any substance or addictive behaviour] – that our lives had become unmanageable.

The essence of the first step is powerlessness. Now, this does not mean the refusal of personal responsibility. It does mean that our egoic efforts are not equipped to deal with addictive substances/behaviour. The addicted subject doesn't control whatever substance he is addicted to – it controls him. We need to rearrange our thoughts here on the subject and realise that we don't *have* a problem – *we are the problem*. To put it bluntly, the ego is a false-self system, giving us a fallacious sense of authorship and ownership. Step One encourages the participant to surrender the operating system of the ego because truly it is not in charge. If I say, 'I am in control of some things and not in control over other things', this means, ultimately, that I am not in control. The Big Book simply starts with: 'Here are the Steps we took which are suggested as a program for recovery' (*Alcoholics Anonymous*, p. 59). Addicted people begin the

DOI: 10.4324/9781003422570-7

journey by acknowledging how unmanageable their lives have become, how they have, perhaps, spun out of control. Advaita too suggests an itinerary to follow; it's called *sadhana* meaning 'the path to accomplishing something'. It's a set of spiritual exercises. Every spiritual discipline possesses one and they all begin with an admission of honest, humble confession/concession: The 'I' that I think I am is not in control of my life.

Step Two

Came to believe that a Power greater than ourselves could restore us to sanity.

In Advaita, the Power in question is the Self – the Absolute. The aim of both the Twelve Steps and Advaita is to enable the person to find his inner Power/Presence. The solution to addiction resides in the power of the Self not the paltry ego ('a tattered coat upon a stick', as W. B. Yeats described it in *Sailing to Byzantium*). Here, we realise that we have a problem we can't fix with our own power, with a mighty will. The ego was dealt a blow in Step One; now comes the reminder that it doesn't run the show – the Self is ultimately in control/charge. To shift gears and transition from ego to Self restores us to sanity. Previously we were 'insane', not clinically so, but in terms of Einstein's famous definition: repeating the same things over and over while looking for a different result. 'This time things will be different', we say, and they never are. For Advaita, insanity is delusion, mistake, ignorance. It's the level we live at when we erroneously think the ego is the real Self. It's to be out of step with the way things actually are.

Exercise: Take a sheet of paper, turn it horizontally, then draw a line across its centre. This is the timeline of your life. At the beginning of the line, write the word 'birth' and then begin to chronologically list significant events of your life. If you consider them to be positive, write them above the line (the more positive they were, the higher above the line you write them) and if you consider them to be negative, write them below the line (the worse they were, the farther below you would write them). Do this right up to the present moment. When completed, look at the role that circumstance played in your life.

Positive
Birth _____
Negative

There is something else at work, something subtler which we can call 'consciousness'. It is a power greater than your egoic self. We can't comprehend that Power. The Big Book follows traditional religion in calling it 'God'. Advaita calls it the Self within which is the divine *Ātman*. From about the age of two (the terrible twos), this *Ātman* is covered up or over through various sheaths that have accrued over time, which obstructs the Self from shining. We begin to see ourselves as separated, independent, isolated individuals, as waves in the ocean rather than the ocean itself, as parts rather than wholes. Each droplet of the ocean contains the entire ocean. Ocean, in this analogy, is essence, consciousness, unity. (There can't be everything plus me over here separate from everything else!) We lose contact with the source, the living centre, over time. Pain and suffering become established. If pain can be seen in terms of not liking what's happening, suffering comes from the feeling that what is happening should not be happening. If pain is a reaction, suffering is a projection.

Step Three

Made a decision to turn our will and our lives over to the care of God as we understand Him.

Do our decisions cause actions? Here, we decide to carry out the will of the Absolute, but this will is nothing other than our Self. So, it is goodness and altruism itself. We are already in the care of the Absolute – it's just that we have lost sight of this truth. We become content with the way things are, recognising there are forces at play outside our control. What is the use in fighting it? The will of the Absolute presents itself as facts of life, frequently as 'blows of fate'. Carrying out the will of the Absolute ultimately means alignment with one's true nature. For example, the sacrifice in love is to surrender to the will of the Absolute. There is a pattern established in the will of the Absolute which forms the very nature of beings – the law of *dharma*, the universal law (more on that anon).

As the ego diminishes, a fuller energy emerges, a new power flows through the being. It is transpersonal in that it is experienced within the personal, but its ultimate origin lies outside and is greater than the purely personal. Consciousness is a universal power. My self-will is the ultimate illusion. Proceeding by the will and way of the Absolute is to follow the nature of being itself. In so far as we don't override this pattern, one lives naturally by universal law and therefore in harmony with oneself and all others too (the Self-same). Love is precisely such a surrendering to 'the will of the Absolute'. If our attachments are strong, then we are cut off from this source of love and we 'go it alone', which is the cause of much misery and mayhem. Selfishness inevitably leads to discontentment. In all situations, we should seek to surrender to the will of the Absolute, for the Self is supereminent, to which the ego is subordinate. Indeed, the main effort of the imperial ego is to overextend itself. In meditation, which is a work of devotion, we focus our attention on the centre. By so doing, we also surrender to the will of the Absolute, because meditation is the movement into the realm of one's Self. Meditation seeks nothing for itself, not even grace. It leads to the being of the Self (the immanent-transcendent Absolute).

Step Four

Made a searching and fearless moral inventory of ourselves.

An inventory of ourselves consists in an examen, not just of conscience but of consciousness itself. Here, we fall still to take stock of the building blocks of our lives. It is the reflective practice of sifting. Business talks of a SWOT analysis: Strengths, Weaknesses, Obstacles/Opportunities, and Threats. The obstacle is the opportunity. In particular, we explore our relationships, our selfishness, dishonesty, resentment, and fears. 'Resentment is like drinking poison and then hoping it will kill your enemies', Nelson Mandela observed. Step Four is our autobiography.

The areas of particular emphasis are resentments, fears, sex, and guilt. It may seem overwhelming or even impossible at first, but keeping a daily journal and being frank becomes easier over time. 'Little and often' is the motto and mantra here. It is about what you consider good and bad, right and wrong. One doesn't take an inventory of others. When we examine the conditions of our lives, we ask what caused or contributed to them. We stay close to our experience. Honesty is humility – it is recognising the truth of what is (not what our minds do with what is). Truth is the conformity of the mind with reality (not the other way around, as stated earlier).

What am I like? What are my characteristics, my sexual nature, my assets, my fears, my rages, and my resentments? What have I done to others and what have others done to me? The inventory is a catalogue of how we relate to others, events, and ourselves, both the positive and the problematic. What is the ultimate source of our behaviour? This is the realm which Advaita adds. It is Self-enquiry and asks, who am I in truth? We spot the patterns, gather together the disparate threads of the tapestry. This is inner work that requires great courage.

Firstly, review your *resentments* – your indignations, which the Big Book says is the number one offender. It is important to note that acceptance is not the same as approval. Secondly, review your *fears*. Thirdly, review your *sexuality*, which is the area and arena in life where there is the greatest chance for deception. Fourthly, explore your feelings of *guilt* and *shame*.

Step Five

Admitted to God, to ourselves, and to another human being the exact nature of our wrongs.

Step Five completes Step Four. This fifth step encourages one to share the information and insights from Step Four with a trusted confidante. It aims to relieve the sense of isolation. One shares one's secrets and by so doing is 'cleansed' – a clearing takes place. Talking is therapeutic; sharing is caring. There is a freedom to be found in disclosure with no disclaimers.

Steps Six and Seven

Were entirely ready to have God remove all these defects of character.

(Step Six)

Humbly asked Him to remove our shortcomings.

(Step Seven)

If a characterological defect is something that is present and can be recognised, a shortcoming is a quality that is absent and not so quickly detected. These steps continue to acknowledge one's personal powerlessness. Note: the person is not asked to do the work of removing these personality impediments. Rather, he/she supplicates the Infinite Unknown, the source and substance of everything to do so. It is petition that requires the virtue of humility and openness.

Steps Eight and Nine

Made a list of all persons we had harmed and became willing to make amends to them all.

(Step Eight)

Made direct amends to such people wherever possible, except when to do so would injure them or others.

(Step Nine)

Here, it is best to first consult with someone before you approach your list of people to make amends in order to plan it out and prepare properly before-hand. Deliberation and forethought are needed. The Promises (as they are called) are enumerated in the Big Book as follows:

- We are going to know a new freedom and a new happiness.
- We will not regret the past nor wish to shut the door on it.
- We will comprehend the word serenity and we will know peace.
- No matter how far down the scale we have gone, we will see how our experience can benefit others.
- That feeling of uselessness and self-pity will disappear.
- We will lose interest in selfish things and gain interest in our fellows.
- Self-seeking will slip away.
- Our whole attitude and outlook upon life will change.
- Fear of people and of economic insecurity will leave us.
- We will intuitively know how to handle situations which used to baffle us.
- We will suddenly realise that God is doing for us what we could not do for ourselves.

(*Alcoholics Anonymous*, pp. 83–84)

The two aspects of resolve are effort and determination. Making amends is making up. It is the restoration of justice and a reconstitution of one's being.

Step Ten

Continued to take personal inventory and when we were wrong promptly admitted it.

Here arrogance is abrogated, and one's faults and failings are admitted. The work of incremental improvement progresses, never ceases. We are works in progress. We don't dwell on wrongs done nor do we procrastinate in recognising them and bringing them into the light. We face our shadow side firmly with fortitude and without flinching.

Step Eleven

Sought through prayer and meditation to improve our conscious contact with God as we understood Him, praying only for knowledge of His will for us and the power to carry that out.

One is enjoined to deliberately set aside some time for both prayer and meditation, praying *only* that we may come to know the will of the Absolute and the power to live that truth – the law of our own being once aligned with our true Self.

As we go through the day we pause, when agitated or doubtful, and ask for the right thought or action. We constantly remind ourselves we are no longer running the show, humbly saying to ourselves many times each day 'Thy will be done'. We are then in much less danger of excitement, fear, anger, worry, self-pity, or foolish decisions. We become much more efficient. We do not tire so easily, for we are not burning up energy foolishly as we did when we were trying to arrange life to suit ourselves.

(*Alcoholics Anonymous*, pp. 87–88)

'Thy will' is always being carried out when we live from the spacious centre of the Self because we live from awareness; we *are* awareness/observers/witnesses. The ego-entity plays its part, but the Self, let us repeat, must direct the symphony. We don't make claims. We recognise that all is the will of the Absolute. Consciousness flows through creation. 'To some extent we have become God-conscious' (*Alcoholics Anonymous*, p. 85). We are not independent actors but manifested forms of the divine Flow of Presence. We are slowly detaching, disidentifying from the false self and finding our fixed abode in the true Self – our inner citadel/interior castle.

True prayer is prayer of the heart rather than petitionary prayer. Prayer is for providence; it creates a space for grace to enter. Everything is already provided. True prayer simply sheds light on that hidden, dormant, universal power in the soul. Meditation is internal, a movement into the Self where there are no thoughts or prayers. Meditation seeks nothing, not even grace. It is union with the cause and centre of all and leads to the being of the Self, the ultimate treasure.

'God grant me the serenity to accept the things I cannot change, the courage to change the things I can, and the wisdom to know the difference' ('Serenity Prayer'). This threefold process (acceptance, change, and knowledge) gets to the nub of the matter. We do this one thought at a time. The Power that has created us has created the world as well. Creation is in the care of the Absolute. On our way, the support of like-minded individuals dedicated and devoted to the Truth will be crucial. Such a spiritual community and gathering is called a *Satsang* in Sanskrit.

Step Twelve

Having had a spiritual awakening as the result of these Steps, we tried to carry this message to alcoholics, and to practice these principles in all our affairs.

We wake up from our previous existence like the prisoners emerging from the shadows of Plato's cave into the sunlight. We become missioned to relay this message of meaning and hope to those who are similarly suffering. We also continue to practice the principles set out above in daily life. A rich tradition of sponsorship/mentorship has developed within the various twelve-step commu-nities/fellowships. Ultimately our words that reflect our thoughts must seep into our actions as we embody/exemplify the teachings and in so doing become living torches of Truth.

Centering Prayer, Contemplative Practice, and the Twelve Steps

I draw here on two well-known American spiritual teachers who have written on the Twelve Steps: Father Thomas Keating, a Cistercian monk and one of the principal developers of 'Centering Prayer' (a term possibly originating with Thomas Merton), a contemporary method of contemplative meditation which draws on the fourteenth-century classic *The Cloud of Unknowing*; and Richard Rohr, a Franciscan friar and founder of the Center for Action and Contempla-tion in New Mexico.

In *Divine Therapy and Addiction*, Keating discusses the relationship between the Twelve Steps and Centering Prayer, with an anonymous alcoholic named Tom S. Both the Twelve Steps and Centering Prayer are spiritual rather than religious programmes. Neither are affiliated to any particular denomination even if both emerged from the Christian tradition. Tom S. observes that 'a growing number of us in A.A. use Centering Prayer to accomplish the meditation requirement in the eleventh step' (Keating, *Divine Therapy and Addiction*, p. 3). Hence, its relevance here to our discussion.

Step One

This step acknowledges that we are all wounded from early childhood and carry these traumatic traces with us unconsciously. We seek the gratification of three needs:

1   Survival and security
2   Affection, esteem, and approval
3   Power and control

Then, from four to eight years of age, the socialisation period takes place, and this intensifies our growing attachment to the gratification of our emotional programmes that become veritable energy centres around which our thoughts, feelings, and desires circulate. The child has identified happiness with the gratification of these three instinctual emotional needs, but reality doesn't meet them (the pleasure principle locks horns with the reality principle) and this contributes to a growing sense of frustration in the child. Some factors incline us to these programmes for 'happiness':

• Temperament
• Biological inheritance
• Number on the Enneagram
• Social conditions

Many carry these residual frustrations with them into adulthood and turn to drinking or drugs to relieve the pain, especially of feelings of rage, rejection, or resentment. The problem is we overidentify with emotional programmes, thinking that the gratification of desires will bring happiness. There are two things wrong here: first, they don't and second, they can't. The reason why many people who have achieved recovery develop another addiction or fall back into the previous addiction is that they carry this fantasy with them in their unconscious. Ongoing daily spiritual practice is a requisite because diminishing the force of this fantasy and falsehood takes time. The Twelve Steps are a path to freedom from compulsions; they are helpful for those with any addiction. The key point that Keating wishes to draw our attention to is that there are deep-rooted unconscious emotional causes and attachments behind addictive behaviour which need to be released, and the emotional programmes for happiness need to be dismantled. He labels this process 'the unloading of the unconscious'. The first step of every serious spiritual journey is to acknowledge that we are powerless, in other words, when helpless/overwhelmed we turn to a higher/deeper Power/Presence. Letting go (surrender) is a movement into freedom. But old patterns are seductive and revisit us in the form of what Freud called 'the return of the repressed', hence, the importance of continual vigilance. The powerlessness resulting from repeated defeat in this process can lead to despair. Attachments to emotional programmes for happiness are deeply embedded in us. We all have hidden addictions, Keating contends. An addiction provides a way of forgetting intolerable pain, if only momentarily. The first step will recognise the reality of our compulsive–addictive desires, our overidentification with the perceived happiness that derives from the gratification of our instinctual needs, and the fact that we are constitutionally self-centred (at the level of the ego-personality). It should also be reiterated that recovery is not limited to people who have an identifiable addiction. It pertains to addicted humanity *per se*. (And I write as one who has not experienced either addiction in the prevailing clinical sense of the term or the Twelve Steps.)

What the New Testament calls 'salvation', and Eastern philosophy calls 'enlightenment', A.A. calls 'recovery'. The central message is the same: transformation into the divine. In *Breathing Under Water: Spirituality and the Twelve Steps*, Richard Rohr says in relation to this first step that the experience of powerlessness is where we all must start (Rohr, *Breathing Under Water*, p. xvii). He begins his book by making four assumptions about addiction (Rohr, *Breathing Under Water*, pp. xxii–xxiv):

1   We are all addicts.
2   'Stinking thinking' is the universal addiction.
3   All societies are addicted to themselves and create deep co-dependency on them.
4   Some form of alternative consciousness is the only freedom from this self and from cultural lies.

In accord with Keating, Rohr asserts that the primary spiritual path must be some form of contemplative practice – a change in our operating system. 'Power is best in weakness' (St Paul, 2 *Corinthians* 12: 9–10) – such is the power of powerlessness. What has to dissolve is the rigid, arrogant, overgrown ego. It is, in reality, too small and selfish to help us. 'The ego defines itself by its attachments' (Rohr, *Breathing Under Water*, p. 5). Spirituality, by contrast, is about letting go.

Step Two

We need to distinguish 'God' from our idea of God. The latter so often pertains to a childhood conception we inherit of a big being (anthropocentrism) in the sky (dualism). The Absolute transcends all conceptions. 'Turning to' the Absolute requires the practice of meditation as it provides a resting in this divine presence which is found in flowers no less than fields and faces. Indeed, all creation 'is permeated by a presence that transcends our sensible faculties' (Keating, *Divine Therapy and Addiction*, p. 20). We don't have to identify the

Higher Power, though, with the God of our childhood. What we call God is not a being (object) but the Ground of Being Itself – the immanent ineffable One.

Over a period of time, we will feel the old cravings return, but they will not be as compulsive as before. The 'human condition' is one that Keating has described as a universal experience whereby we unconsciously act as if our happiness is going to occur as the result of the gratification of our instinctual needs. 'Faith' or 'trust' is the religious equivalent of 'letting go'. We need to admit that we have such enormous amounts of investment in worldly objectives/objects of desire. Our childhood emotional programmes are still with us in our unconscious or 'heart' (innermost being). We recycle them over and over. Let's begin by conceding this truth. There are three consequences of the human condition:

1   Illusion (not knowing where true happiness lies)
2   Concupiscence (looking for happiness in all the wrong places, or too much in the right places)
3   Weakness of the will, *akrasia* (even if we do find where true happiness is, our will is too weak to do anything about it)

'Repentance' is one name from within the religious register to denote a profound change or conversion in the direction in which we are looking for happiness. Rohr describes three inner openings (Rohr, *Breathing Under Water*, pp. 10–12):

1   The mind space – to keep the mind open we need some form of contemplative practice (nondual consciousness).
2   The heart space – here we need healing from past hurts and horrors. The Enneagram is one 'marvellous spiritual tool that names the nine most common "programs for happiness" or strategies for survival' (p. 11).
3   The body space – to keep our bodies less defended by being present to people in a cellular way (the body never lies).

The work of spirituality is an ongoing liberation of heart, head, and body. For Rohr, the Presence is the Highest Power. 'May the God of peace make you whole and holy, may you be kept safe in body, heart, and mind, and thus ready for the presence' (St Paul, 1 *Thessalonians* 5: 23).

Step Three

Keating recommends, with A.A., conscious contact with the Absolute (universal consciousness) for 20–30 minutes twice daily, once in the morning and once in the evening, 'in the silence of centering prayer' (Keating, *Divine Therapy and Addiction*, p. 40), because we are all recovering from something, and we need divine psychotherapy. The kingdom of heaven is a state of consciousness.

Keating describes meditation as a 'healing practice' (Keating, *Divine Therapy and Addiction*, p. 74). The quietening of the mind leads to the experience of peace in the psyche. This, in turn, results in the reduced demand for the emotional programmes for happiness to be satisfied. Our inner blockage to 'turning things over' (namely, our will-to-power) is overcome by an existential decision. Our primary addiction is to our own power and false programmes for happiness. 'If anyone wants to follow me, let him renounce himself' (*Mark* 8: 34; *Luke* 9: 23; *Matthew* 16: 4). Renunciation of ego is what Bill W means in Step Three by the radical surrender of our will.

Step Four

The inventory is the taking of a life-history, which requires both humility and honesty. Pride is insidious. We survey our conduct, paying particular attention to sex, security, and society. Keating notes: 'The spiritual journey is going in the same direction as AA and involves the same essential Steps' (Keating, *Divine Therapy and Addiction*, p. 52). Keating encourages all those on the Twelve Steps to return to the truth of their basic goodness as human beings. Holistic health is the goal of all therapy and spiritual direction, as well as the Twelve Steps.

'Compunction' is the name given to the sadness produced from seeing one's failures and weaknesses. But, as Rohr suggests, people come to deeper consciousness only through crises, contradictions, conflicts, and confusions – what religion calls 'sin' (see Rohr, *Breathing Under Water*, p. 31). The ego is intent on denying or denouncing such shadow material. 'Evil proceeds from a lack of consciousness' (Rohr, *Breathing Under Water*, p. 35). To observe the splinter in my brother's eyes means noticing the plank in my own.

What can also be included in this fourth step is a Japanese structured and specific method of self-reflection known as *Naikan*, which is rooted in Asian philosophy. Developed by the Japanese Buddhist Yoshimoto Ishin, *Naikan* means 'inside looking' (introspection); it is seeing with the mind's eye. Over forty centres in Japan, and some too in Austria and Germany, offer *Naikan* (which complements Morita therapy). The process can be used in counselling, addiction recovery, and rehabilitation programmes in prisons. The shift involved is from a zoom lens to a wide-angle lens (a broader panorama/perspective). It is rooted in all the great spiritual traditions, from the Christian mystics to the Japanese samurai. *Naikan* has three components:

1 Time is set aside each day for this self-reflection exercise.
2 A space is used that limits external distractions.
3 The application of questions.

We humans have the capacity for self-reflection, to observe our thoughts and feelings. So, in *Naikan*, we reflect on ourselves and our relationships in a quiet place, asking:

- What have I received from _____?
- What have I given to _____?
- What troubles and difficulties have I caused _____?

We put our attention on what we have received from life/people which elicits gratitude and puts attention on appreciation. Then, we become aware of what we have given to others. Next, we realise our part in their suffering (usually we justify our bad behaviour with 'I didn't mean to', 'it's no big deal', 'it was an accident'). This daily exercise (*Nichijo Naikan*) is done for 20–30 minutes before bedtime, and we write down the answers to the questions (journaling). One can do a longer version and explore the last few years of their life or engage in this contemplative practice in a week's retreat (*Shuchu Naikan*) totally secluded. Here, we observe the screen of our lives, which is based on a script – not on our ego editing but on the original draft! We simply watch/witness the movie.

Step Five

One admits one's faults to others much like the early Irish monks and Desert Fathers did. *Mea culpa, mea maxima culpa*. This task is much akin to confession. An increase in inner freedom is the result, as the person implicated in the process moves from shame to loving acceptance. Humility is nothing other than acceptance. It is more about selfless respect for reality than the habit of self-effacement and one of the most central and difficult of all the virtues. This step points to accountability and personal responsibility. The Twelve Steps believes that the arena of failure is the perfect opportunity for the enlightenment of the offender. We can distinguish between two juridical systems:

- Retributive justice
- Restorative justice

The former has been the prevailing model for centuries and operates against the backdrop of punishment, whereas the latter revolutionary programme responds to crime through dialogue and reconciliation. If the former has an economy of merit as its central message based on a relationship of *quid pro quo*, the latter proceeds by way of an economy of grace. It is love rather than law that effects true inner transformation. Rohr describes these two patterns thus (Rohr, *Breathing Under Water*, p. 42):

sin → punishment → repentance → transformation : ego

sin → unconditional love → transformation → repentance : Self

In Catholicism, the sacrament of confession is the accountability system. In times of doubt and darkness, we need an *anamchara* (as we say in Ireland) or soul-friend. At this sixth stage, the necessity for peer confession or counselling comes into play to restore communion and natural harmony. If we don't engage with apology and forgiveness, then we are controlled by our past. Rohr calls them 'the divine technology for the regeneration of every age' (Rohr, *Breathing Under Water*, p. 49).

Steps Six and Seven

We hanker after happiness but have no idea really where it is to be found. This lack of knowing – our mistaken beliefs around this – is *maya*. Our emotional life begins in the womb. We fallaciously interpret the gratification of our instinctual needs as happiness. The more our three instinctual needs are not met, the more we suffer from trauma. These undigested emotional experiences (stored in the body) accompany us throughout life. They represent the full gamut of unmet needs from rage to resentment. Over time, the child begins to build what Keating calls a 'homemade self' (Keating, *Divine Therapy and Addiction*, p. 71). It's false because it responds to the emotional programmes for happiness that the child first formulated/formatted in early life. In the sixth step, we become willing for our faults to be cured (willingness is not willpower). Our faults/failings won't disappear through our existential efforts alone – but 'God willing' (grace). 'Our emotional programs for happiness are never going to work' (Keating, *Divine Therapy and Addiction*, p. 82). The false-self system is responsible for much of our fear, misery, and illusion-making. The ego's imaginings are not congruent with that which is/the way things are.

Turning our will over to God is the beginning of the undoing of fear together with the false-self system. (And here we should be mindful of our speech, taking care we say 'I've *feelings* of fear' rather than 'I'm afraid'). The beginnings of attachment are the identification of the 'I' with an activity or feeling, etc. 'The real you is the great "I am", the center of our being, the Source from which we emerge, body, soul, and spirit', writes Keating (Keating, *Divine Therapy and Addiction*, p. 86). In this context, Keating describes and defines addiction as 'the last resort of the psyche to avoid unbearable pain' (Keating, *Divine Therapy and Addiction*, p. 86). Anyone who hasn't engaged in the work of dismantling the false self will acquire an addiction of some sort. The constant mental chatter and commentary on our feelings lead to 'emotional binges' (Keating, *Divine Therapy and Addiction*, p. 90). It's basically a takeover of the human brain by the reptilian or mammalian brain. Repeating a formula can help here, such as: 'O God, come to my aid, O Lord, make haste to help me', which was a favourite of the Desert Fathers and appears in the writings of John Cassian. The sacred word is said, then sounded – interiorised. Of all the obstacles and impediments (defence mechanisms, in the language of psychoanalysis), perhaps the greatest is thinking too much. Meditation is about not thinking; it's about being out of one's mind. And one doesn't have to wait for a set period of meditation to do this. When, for example, fear arises, one drops it as fast as possible; one starves it of oxygen by depriving it of attention. Keating's 'welcoming prayer' is deployed. We welcome everything that comes to us – all thoughts, emotions, persons, situations. We let go of the desire for power and control, for affection and approval, for survival and security. We surrender the desire to change the situation. We submit to the will of the Absolute (in the language of Vedanta). And open to the Presence within. This can be done in a moment, in a breath. It is acceptance of what is and needed because 'everybody is in the addictive process' (Keating, *Divine Therapy and Addiction*, p. 88). The emotional programmes for happiness are actually programmes for ill health – they are worsened with and warped by commentary. Meditation enables us to disidentify from our thoughts. Now, meditation can make us more vulnerable (especially during long intensive periods of meditation such as retreats) to primitive undigested emotional material – to bombardments of unwanted thoughts deriving from the unconscious, but we disregard this unloading of the unconscious by returning to the mantra or sacred word. The divine therapy of meditation does its healing work regardless. Of course, there are times when psychological help will have to be sought. There is, after all, a dimensional difference between a clinical depression and a dark night of the sense or spirit *à la* St John of the Cross. The aim is the emptying of ego (*kenosis*). The ego extracted from its source in the Self will experience either:

- Exaltation when its instinctual needs are gratified (the emotional programmes for happiness).
- Frustration/depression when such needs are not met.

In Bill W's case, as we can glean from his correspondence with the Jesuit Father Dowling, he had a depression for over twelve years and couldn't get rid of it precisely because it was rooted in an emotional programme from the past. In time, he saw that he was a people-pleaser – he was invested in that particular emotional programme. *Underlying his addiction to alcohol was the need for approval.* 'Alcoholics need to realise that underneath their addiction to alcohol is a deeper problem' (Keating, *Divine Therapy and Addiction*, p. 97). Divine therapy is slow but steadfast. By contrast, 'If you just take chemicals, all that you cure are the symptoms' (Keating, *Divine Therapy and Addiction*, p. 106). Psychiatry only treats the body and the brain. The human being is more than a clump of cells or chemicals, so much more than a mere mass of molecules. 'The purpose of the divine therapy is the healing of the roots of all our problems and to transform our attitudes' (Keating, *Divine Therapy and Addiction*, p. 107). That is why the Twelve Steps of A.A. 'addresses the whole person – body, soul, and spirit' (Keating, *Divine Therapy and Addiction*, p. 110) precisely because it is a spiritual programme, one with contemplation at its core. 'Letting go of attachment to finding happiness in one of those three basic instinctual needs is the radical road to recovery and human health' (Keating, *Divine Therapy and Addiction*, p. 113). It is not, however, enough to recover from addiction – one must also recover from the addictive process itself. Centering Prayer's (and this is only one method and option) aim is to provide the contemplative conditions for communing with the Absolute and cultivating interior silence. A practice of meditation could be more formally introduced in the third step rather than waiting until the eleventh, Keating opines.

'If I will it? Of course I will it! Be healed' (*Luke* 5: 12). Resistances are removed through surrender ('Let it be done unto me'; *Luke* 23: 46). One ancient aphorism goes thus: we pray as if all depends on us and nothing on the Absolute, and we work as if it all depends on the Absolute and nothing on us. We petition not to change the Absolute but ourselves. We thus become poor in spirit, powerless, mendicants. By so doing, the scaffolding of the constructed small self dismantles and diminishes.

Step Eight

Parents can do much harm to their children through their inadequacy or by their intentional or inadvertent emotional deficits. The addicted parent is not present psychically to their child, even if they are present physically. If, later on, the addicted subject is unable to forgive them, resentment can set in. Making amends is to forgive, and forgiveness comes from the heart; it melts the bars of resentment and is another path to inner freedom. One is forgiven only after one has forgiven.

This is the stage of reconciliation, restoration. We 'transcend and include' our former way of life. Earlier wrongs are rectified. The *karma* of past mistakes can catch us up, so the bonds that have been broken need repair and reconstitution. Rohr stresses the importance here of redemptive listening and non-violent communication (Rohr, *Breathing Under Water*, p. 70). We seek to move beyond our niggardly narcissism. This comes through effort and amazing grace, in the Christian tradition; in other words, both axes of the cross are required – the vertical and the horizontal dimensions (sacred geometry). We 'become' willing, so it is a process that can't be rushed. The heart gradually softens, and our attachments loosen. We make a list, not of those who have hurt us, but of those whom we have mistreated. Einstein's advice is apposite: no problem can be solved by the same consciousness that caused the problem in the first place.

Step Nine

One consults with one's sponsor and/or spiritual director, which is an additional resource, before proceeding to make amends with different persons. If met with indignation or outrage, the person will need to recover a bit first before setting out again. We are responsible only for our efforts – never for the results. What is needed is good judgement/discernment, a careful sense of timing, courage, and prudence. If the person in question is deceased, one can always pray for them (the purpose of which is to effect a change in us) or perform a ritual, such as lighting a candle, for them. Step Nine insists that we use skilful means to make amends; these should be specific, personal, and concrete. Context is paramount.

Step Ten

Living in the present mindfully is the answer to worrying (future) and reminiscing (past). The former can become anticipatory anxiety and the latter a melancholic dwelling. Being in the moment detaches us from our unconscious motivation so that we aren't as dominated by emotions and thoughts. Rather, we experience the deep rest of contemplative living – from a place of response rather than reaction.

The examen of *conscience* was later changed to the examen of *consciousness*. This method of meditation was popularised by the Jesuit Order. Rohr describes consciousness thus: 'Consciousness is not the seeing but *that which sees me seeing*. It is not the knower but *that which knows that I am knowing*. It is not the observer but *that which underlies and observes me observing*' (Rohr, *Breathing Under Water*, p. 85). Consciousness is aware of my feelings so it cannot simply be my feelings themselves. Availing of/becoming the true Self is to put on 'the mind of Christ' (Christic consciousness; 1 *Corinthians* 2: 10–16) in the language of Rohr's Christian formulations on the subject (albeit from a nondual perspective). The Spirit is the Advocate (*John* 14: 16) who is 'with you and in you' (*John* 14: 17). This is the Self of Advaita, the *Ātman*, the secret inner Source. Due to the fact that consciousness has become unconscious, it is no wonder, according to Rohr, that we try to fill this 'radical disconnectedness' with various addictions (Rohr, *Breathing Under Water*, p. 88). God, in this understanding, is 'Universal Consciousness' (Rohr, *Breathing Under Water*, p. 91).

Step Eleven

Contemplation proceeds by way of a movement from concentration to receptivity. What Eastern philosophy means by 'meditation', Christian spirituality means by 'contemplation'. Throughout his works, Keating distinguishes between *two* forms or facets/faces of the unconscious (Keating, *Divine Therapy and Addiction*, p. 152):

- Psychological
- Ontological

One way of understanding 'the unconscious' is viewing it as an energy system that dwells in people as a result of repressed trauma. If the psychological unconscious is understood along classic Freudian lines, the ontological unconscious refers to the level of being. The collective unconscious, for Jung, designates the shared experience of the human race (phylogenesis). So, it is the unconscious presence of absolute consciousness made conscious that is the end of the Twelve Steps. The whole purpose of the Twelve Steps is to become conscious of the presence of the Absolute (God-Self) – the unity of *Ātman* with *Brahman*. 'The Divine Indwelling is a loving presence of God within us' (Keating, *Divine Therapy and Addiction*, p. 152). According to Keating, one becomes rooted in the three theological virtues of faith, hope, and charity; the four infused virtues of temperance, courage, justice, and practical wisdom; and the nine fruits of the Holy Spirit (charity, joy, peace, gentleness, self-constraint, patience, goodness, generosity, and faithfulness); as well as the seven gifts of the Spirit (wisdom, understanding, counsel, fortitude, knowledge, piety, and fear of the Lord). These qualities are manifestations of our true Self, as expressed in the Christian tradition. Meditation opens us to the Ultimate Reality. Over time, 'one begins to lose interest in the addictive process or in the addiction' (Keating, *Divine Therapy and Addiction*, p. 156). Exposure to silence offers universal healing. A spiritual awakening is a Self-awakening into an expanded state of consciousness.

'Be still and know that I am God' (*Psalms* 46: 10). Prayer and meditation are code words for an entirely different way of processing life, Rohr contends (Rohr, *Breathing Under Water*, p. 94). We put on a different 'thinking cap' and move from a calculative mind to a contemplative mind. Meditation can be described as 'an alternative processing system' (Rohr, *Breathing Under Water*, p. 95), one that involves a positive widening of one's lens to get a better picture, an emptying of the mind and a filling of the heart. I thus draw from the Deeper Well. '*The small mind cannot deal with Bigness and Newness*' (Rohr, *Breathing Under Water*, p. 97). Rohr calls meditation '*the prayer of quiet*' (Rohr, *Breathing Under Water*, p. 98), one which heals the unconscious, in complete accord with Keating.

Step Twelve

Keating makes the plea that Centering Prayer be introduced into A.A. as part of its programme so that it can become a *contemplative* twelve-step programme. What's important is that those following the Twelve Steps meditate, so the discipline of meditation could be introduced at the third or sixth step at least, but it is explicitly recommended/required in the twelfth step. We can detect two discernible movements within a meditation:

1 The unloading of the unconscious (release of repressed material)
2 The transformation of consciousness (as we gradually grow into divinity – *theosis*)

(Of course, it is not I who am divine but the Spirit within.) The analogy is the change from being a caterpillar to a butterfly. The 'Higher Power' is none other than the Absolute. Relating to this may involve any of the following meditative measures:

- Reading sacred scriptures (*lectio divina*) or the words of the wise (philosophy)
- Reflecting/ruminating (examen of consciousness)
- Responding (to the divine Pull) in thoughts, words, and deeds
- Resting (abiding in the Presence of the Most High who is also our Deepest Self and availing of sustainable happiness)

The indwelling Trinity (*sat–chit–ananda*: being–consciousness–bliss) heals the wounds of our humanity. In time, there will be preferences with no addiction and desire with no attachment. And then our distress will transmogrify into delight.

'What was given to you freely, you must give away freely' (*Matthew* 10: 8). This final step summons one to loving service. In this regard, Rohr reminds us of the first law of thermodynamics: energy cannot be created or destroyed; it is merely converted to different uses. What comes around, goes around (see Rohr, *Breathing Under Water*, p. 109). It brings one back to where we should all start – with the necessity of a spiritual awakening. Awakening is the Great Change, the change that changes everything. Rohr concludes his book *Breathing Under Water* with several observations (Rohr, *Breathing Under Water*, pp. 115–117):

- Addiction is a spiritual dis-ease.
- Addictions are the result of frustrated desire.
- Addicts tend to confuse intensity with intimacy.
- Addiction is idolatry (absolutizing what is only of relative value).
- We're all compulsive consumers and shouldn't waste any more time on worshipping gods that can't save us.
- The addict has taken a wrong turn.
- More and more of anything just doesn't work.

Chapter 7

The Hero's Journey

Myths

The question is, where to start on the journey and what might it look like? The Hero's Journey outlines some archetypal steps for us. *Our self is storied.* We each live out a 'personal myth', and so we must consider these dimensions of the human personality if our attempts to bring about change are to be effective and lasting. My personal myth will be the central story behind the various episodes of my life, which are happenings whose impact is profound because they operate largely outside my conscious awareness. It is the story I have for making sense and meaning of the world, the story I am living.

In terms of mythology, the torments of Tantalus are the addicted subject's, who has yet to find his desire stuck, as he is, in *jouissance*. According to this Greek myth, Tantalus was welcomed to Zeus's table, but stole ambrosia and nectar, revealed the secrets of the gods, committed perjury, and killed his son and served him as a meal to the gods. His punishment – now a proverbial term for *temptation without satisfaction* ('to tantalise') – was to stand in the river Eridanos beneath fruit trees with low branches. Whenever he reached for the fruit, the branches raised it from his grasp, and whenever he bent down to get a drink, the water receded before he could get any.

Before exploring the Hero's Journey and its applicability to addiction, let's say something briefly about the form and function of myths first. Myths are stories of our search through the ages for truth, meaning, and significance. Through myths we touch the eternal. Joseph Campbell, the famous mythologist, changed the definition of a myth from the *search* for meaning to the *experience* of meaning. Myths bring messages – they are stories about the wisdom of life. Mythology is the song of the imagination. A myth is a story about the gods. A god is a personification of a motivating power or value system. The mystical function of a myth is to realise what a wonder the universe is – we marvel at mystery. What comes out in myths is the following: at the bottom of the abyss in the journey inward is the voice of salvation. The black moment of despair, which all addicted persons can relate to, is when the real message of

DOI: 10.4324/9781003422570-8

transformation occurs. Three symbols spring up: that of the serpent which is bound to earth and that of the eagle which designates spiritual flight. The dragon is the amalgamation of these two forces (a serpent with wings). Myths pertain to both the personal dimension (the work of Freud) and a collective or archetypal dimension (the work of Jung). If the former is biographical, the latter is biological. Dreams correlate with myths. A myth is a public dream, and the dream is a private myth. Myths are to the race what dreams are to the individual. (For an extended discussion of myths, see the following: Joseph Campbell, *The Hero with a Thousand Faces* and *The Power of Myth*; Rollo May, *The Cry for Myth*; Luc Ferry, *The Wisdom of the Myths*; Mark Patrick Hederman, *Living the Mystery*.)

When you interpret metaphors as facts, you're in trouble; this gives rise to literalism. A metaphor is an image that suggests something else. Myth reads the world in terms of poetry (connotation) rather than prose (denotation). Civilisations are grounded on myth and myth is grounded in the unconscious. To deploy three more symbols: the Cathedral (government of the spirit), the Castle (government of physical life), and the Cottage (where the people dwell). Or, to put it another way, the Temple, the Tower, and the Town – different centres all operating in the same symbolic field. Mythographers have been dealing with stories and fairy tales collected over the course of twelve centuries: from the seventh century BC to the fifth century AD. Myth, one could say, is philosophy in story form. Mythology delivers messages of meaning to mortals. Mythologists were the first storytellers. We can adduce four functions of myths (see May, *The Cry for Myth*, pp. 15–29):

1 Myths reveal our prehistory – the origin of the world. They are indispensable for understanding the good life.
2 They ask, how are we mortal men going to insert ourselves into this universe of the gods that does not seem to have been made for mortals? Myths help situate us meaningfully. Life is here seen as a quest or a search for order – for the meaning of our lives (exemplified by and encapsulated in the Hero's Journey).
3 The mismeasure of life is a theme that runs through Greek myth. It's concerned with *hubris* – the choice men make to set themselves up against the divine and cosmic order of the gods. Wisdom is seen as finding your natural place in a divine and everlasting order.
4 We occupy the space between (the middle path or *metaxy*). Ours is human fate and we must face our ordeals, meet monsters from the deep.

The 'gods' always bring us to order. *Cosmos* connotes the harmonious order of things. Its opposite is chaos. *Hubris* – pride – is seen as the greatest vice. It means not knowing our proper place (ourselves), giving rise to discord and resistance. 'KNOW THYSELF!' was the first Delphic dictum. *Dike* – justice – is the greatest virtue. It means being in accord/agreement with cosmic order. NOTH-ING TO EXCESS – in all things moderation (temperance), was the second say-ing, which has obvious lessons in it for all those struggling with addiction.

The major myths deal with *hubris* and *dike*; and the deranged acts of im-moderation perpetrated by certain individuals, as well as other just acts carried out by heroes (who show us how to act properly). *Hubris* involves conflict with the cosmic order that brings the contempt of the gods. We're all on a Hero's Journey like Odysseus as he travels through eleven steps on his way to mortal wisdom, as he journeys from Troy to Ithaca, from war to peace (in Homer's *Odyssey*). *Hubris* is the cosmos menaced by a return to chaos. The absence of wisdom spoils the existence of mortals.

The temple at Delphi was an oracle of wisdom – a celebrated monument raised to the glory of Apollo. Proverbs from Greek wisdom were engraved in the stone, enshrining tenets of practical philosophy. 'Know thyself!' and 'Noth-ing to excess' were adopted by Socrates and later psychologised by Freud. The original meaning: not to get above ourselves/our station, to stay in our allotted place, knowing our limits, not flying off, guarding against arrogance and im-moderation that puts us out of balance, which leads to disaster. Myth is about the measure of man. The great Greek emphasis was always on wholeness/inte-gration. Order is inner harmony; disorder is being out of balance. A myth is a way of making sense of things. *Myths are our way of finding this meaning.* Mythmaking is as essential as meaning-making in gaining mental health. Cults have the power of myths without the social limits. Myths refer to the quintes-sence of human life. Myths give us a sense of personal identity, make possible a sense of community, undergird our moral values, and enable us to deal with the mystery of creation. For example, the existential crisis of work is expressed in the myth of Sisyphus (a modern take on which is F. Scott Fitzgerald's *The Great Gatsby*).

The myth of the homeland is symbolised by the hero who represents our highest aspirations and ideals (someone on a real journey who is struggling and suffering, for example, with an addiction. The Hero's Journey is the ad-dicted person's journey *par excellence*). Our heroes carry our aspirations, ide-als, and hopes. Myths and legends bear in heroicised form our history. Myths are means of discovery (a new reality). Myths deal with pilgrims, pioneers, explorers, travellers. Mythic intelligence is the middle voice between fact and fiction, science, and religion. A mythic-poetic language has all but been lost under the rule of scientific rationalism.

On the one hand, you have the myth of the American dream (the golden touch of King Midas) and on the other hand, you have the myth of Sisyphus which counters the 'American dream'. This myth denies progress and is about endless repetition, perpetual monotonous toil and sweat. But one thing Sisy-phus can do is be aware of each moment of this drama between himself and Zeus, between himself and his fate, as he unsuccessfully pushes his boulder up the hill. His human response is most human. Punished by Zeus for deceiving the gods, Sisyphus is described by Homer thus:

> With many a weary step, and many a groan,
> Up the high hill he heaves a huge round stone;
> The huge round stone, resulting with a bound,
> Thunders impetus down.

This myth is a meditation on monotony. Sisyphus who continues to push the boulder daily knowing he will never topple it over is a hero for our time in his refusal to give up. He is the model of a hero who presses on, in spite of despair and (inner) demons, of alcoholism or addiction. Without such courage and perseverance, the world would not have Beethoven or Rembrandt or Michelangelo, or Dante or Goethe, or any of the great men and women down the centuries.

Sisyphus placed the monotony (the rolling of the stone) in the scheme of his rebellion. Every act of Sisyphus was a revolt against the gods of conformity. Each act was one of penance and purpose, of patience and perseverance. This myth shows us that the meaning of human existence is infinitely deeper than Gatsby's dream and the American dream (the empire of happiness). When 'eternity breaks into time', which they do in myths, we are confronted with all human existence – the tragic and the triumphant aspects. Sisyphus teaches the addicted person and, indeed, all of us how to go on when we don't want to go on throughout our ordeals, as we seek to find meaning (*logos*) in suffering (*pathos*).

The Hero's Journey

The Hero's Journey has the structure of a monomyth. Like the twelve-step programmes, there are twelve stages too in the Hero's Journey. The main character is the Hero (we can see him as one who has overcome his addictions, in our context). It begins with him in one place and ends with him in another (physically and emotionally). The Hero is the same regardless of the story (but he appears in different forms). The paths are different (he may be an accountant or a teacher), but the journey is the same. The Hero will encounter other characters (archetypes) along the way. These could be the Herald, the Mentor, the Goddess, the Trickster. The Hero could be Harry Potter or King Arthur or Frodo – the path is similar. The mentor might be Dumbledore or Merlin or Gandalf; his role is always to guide the hero. This structure appears everywhere (in books and movies). For example, Luke Skywalker leaves his home on Tatooine, has adventures, and fulfils his potential as a Jedi. Joseph Campbell's model proposes seventeen stages, but Christopher Vogler in *The Writer's Journey* elaborates an abbreviated version of twelve, which we will follow here. The dialectic is always remove, receive, return.

The Hero's Journey is drawn from the depth psychology of C. G. Jung and the mythological studies of Joseph Campbell. Vogler suggests: 'the Hero's Journey is nothing less than a handbook for life, a complete instruction manual in the art of being human' (Vogler, *The Writer's Journey*, p. xiii). The hero is a warrior (but that is only one of his/her faces). The hero is also a pilgrim, wanderer, hermit, inventor, artist, clown, king, slave, worker, rebel, adventurer, saint, teacher, nurse. All stories consist of a few common structural elements found universally in fairy tales, dreams, and films. These meaning motifs are *archetypes* (the trickster, wise old man, *puer aeternus*). Archetypes are universal patterns (symbolic images) of the psyche.

'Hero' is a person who takes the lead in the journey. 'Hero' means 'protector' or 'defender' (think of Hector or Heracles). He is a person who performs a service to those in need, defends certain ideals, shows courage in combat, and is celebrated in ancient legends. A hero is wise, strong, reliable, resilient, caring, charismatic, inspiring, selfless. Call these the eight great traits of a hero. Heroes give us wisdom, enhance our lives, provide moral modelling, and offer protection.

The Hero sets out from a comfortable reality (cosy consensus) to venture into the unknown. He faces trials and tribulations, encounters obstacles and opportunities, discovers great treasures, and embarks on a hazardous journey home. Sometimes, the hero is hapless, not even the best person to go on an adventure, but he is willing to embark on a perilous journey. He will grow into the role. (Gilgamesh is arrogant and selfish; Achilles is childish even though an awesome warrior; King Arthur shows no strength before he pulls the sword – Excalibur – from the stone.) They *become* heroic. The Hero is very ordinary. The journey he is on is an opportunity for transformation. The King's role is to protect him and let him go. The Warrior's role is to support the King – he defends the King's interests. The Fool embodies uncomfortable truth.

There are also dragons and demons that test the Hero. His path is well-trodden. For example, Homer, Virgil, Dante, Shakespeare, Milton, James Joyce, as well as in Greek tragedy (Aeschylus) – Prometheus and Zeus (myth was at the centre of fifth-century Athens). The Hero's Journey is a universal story. We can all relate. It begins with implicit threats to the home ground. A crisis calls something into question (e.g., in the *Iliad*, the beautiful Helen is stolen). In Homer's *Odyssey*, Odysseus travels from the Trojan War home to Ithaca. He departs for Troy, then his home descends into anarchy. His city is left without a leader. With somebody at the end of his tether (or his friends and family at the end of theirs) experiencing depression or addiction, the crisis is his low ebb; often it comes as a cry for help, a plea, or suicidal ideation.

Myths pertain to humanity's ancestral attic (the collective unconscious). Myths, legends, and fairy tales point to a Great Escape, to an otherworld beyond our ordinary world, which is one of magic and enchantment and incantations. They have consolation as a core ingredient – the Happy Ending always awaits.

We can summarise the twelve stages of the Hero's Journey under five main themes:

1 *Preparation*: Skill sets, strategies, techniques, and toolkits are manufactured for the task. The Hero sets out on a solitary journey or is accompanied by a fellow traveller or an entire band of brothers (alone or with support;

rehab/A.A., for example). The Guide is a helper to the Hero. He embodies wisdom (an essential characteristic) and usually has access to mythic powers. He may be a magician like Merlin or Gandalf (vision and advice rather than action). The Guide is the therapist, psychologist, or medical team.

2 *Escape*: Often the way out is guarded by a demon or dragon from the depths. Some opponent or obstacle must be overcome, some danger defeated. This is the first challenge (e.g., Jason kills the dragon to get the Golden Fleece; Odysseus fights Cyclops). The Hero fights the guardian of the threshold (to find something he needs). He may get gold or goblets. In his first confrontation, the hero finds his fortitude. He will need courage to continue on this path.

3 *Tests and trials*: The Hero is in a new world; taken from the familiar into the foreign. Obstacles abound. The Hero vacillates between mania and melancholia. A myth has a message, and contains a series of tests, tasks, riddles, puzzles, and pitfalls, which suggests that it's more important to be smart than strong (e.g., in Tolkien's *The Hobbit*, Gollum's puzzle must be answered like the riddles of the Sphinx. Distractions and temptations lure him off course). A successful Hero is steadfast. Sacrifice is part of the journey (Daedalus survives and gets to leave the labyrinth; Icarus dies). The Hero befriends the ugly and rejected, the marginalised and forgotten (in himself first of all – he confronts his shadow, as we all must). Help comes to the Hero from unexpected sources. The lesson: always be open to passing angels (e.g., the frog must be kissed for the prince to find his princess; a toothless hag is the font of wisdom; locked inside Pandora's Box was every evil, disease, and horror, yet hope lurked there too). So don't be dismissive of possible solutions in the unlikeliest of places. The Hero steers the middle ground, avoiding extremes, abrogating arrogance – that he can do this alone, admitting powerlessness. The Middle Way is measure (it's the basis of the ethical philosophy of both Aristotle and the Buddha; e.g., Odysseus navigates between the Scylla/monster and the Charybdis/whirlpool).

4 *Supreme ordeal and reward*: Often overcome by despair or disillusionment, the Hero feels his world turning upside down. He encounters meaninglessness – the dark night of the soul (a near-death experience). Our adventurer experiences Hades rather than Heaven. But if he survives the shipwreck or navigates the waters of the Styx, he will receive his reward. Peace is promised beyond the darkness of desolation. Now the meaning of the journey becomes clear. The elixir comes into sight even if the journey is not quite over. He is well on his way.

5 *Homecoming*: The return journey is also perilous. Rewards can be lost or damaged or seized. (Our unlikely hero might have a relapse.) Dangers lurk – temptations too. There is no guarantee of 'happily ever after'. Even when the Hero returns, he forfeits the freedom he previously enjoyed on his travels (e.g., Orpheus is told not to look back. He does and loses his wife, Eurydice. Oisín returns from the land of eternal youth – Tír na n'Óg – but forgets the conditions of his return and puts his foot on the soil and instantly turns into

an old man and dies). The Hero returns to a strange, changed place to which he must accommodate himself. Time has passed. He will meet with suspicion and hostility (especially from old friends, drinking buddies, fellow addicts). Emissaries may be as formidable as adversaries. Some Heroes are accepted, others rejected, some celebrated, others censored. Nothing can be taken for granted.

The Twelve Stages of the Hero's Journey

The Hero archetype represents the ego in its search for identity, wholeness and meaning, as he/she journeys through the stages of life, to the Self. These are the twelve stages of the Hero's Journey:

1 Ordinary World
2 Call to Adventure
3 Refusal of the Call
4 Meeting with the Mentor
5 Crossing the First Threshold
6 Tests, Allies, Enemies
7 Approach of the Inmost Cave
8 Ordeal
9 Reward
10 The Road Back
11 Resurrection
12 Return with the Elixir

Exercise: As we go through the twelve steps of the Hero's Journey, personalise it, asking yourself how you negotiate(d) and manage(d) the twelve stages and think of examples from your own life to illustrate the process.

There are three acts:

• Act I (Comfort): Ordinary World; Call to Adventure; Refusal of the Call; Mentor; First Threshold; Tests, Allies, Enemies
• Act II (Crisis): Approach to Inmost Cave; Ordeal; Reward
• Act III (Climax): Road Back; Resurrection; Return with the Elixir

To summarise, Act I is about separation. Act IIa is the descent, Act IIb is the initiation, and Act III is the return.

Ordinary World/Home

This is where the Hero exists before his present story begins, oblivious of the adventures (and difficulties) to come. It's his safe place. His everyday, ordinary life is where we learn about him – his nature, outlook, etc. This anchors the

Hero as human (with whom we can identify and empathise, which will become important later; e.g., Dorothy Gale living on her farm in *The Wizard of Oz*.) He may feel boxed in or be snugly/smugly content (e.g., Bilbo Baggins in *The Hobbit*).

Exercise: (You'll need a journal for these.) Reflect on what is familiar, on what you know and love in life. List three things that keep you rooted and make you feel safe/secure. This could be a person, a place, or a principle.

Call to Adventure

The Hero's Journey begins when he receives a call to adventure/action. It usually arrives as a direct threat to his safety or family or way of life. His pernicious peace is disturbed. Something happens, manifests itself (be it a gunshot or conversation or arrival of a stranger), which disrupts his ordinary life and presents him with a challenge or call or quest that must be undertaken (e.g., Harry Potter receives a letter from Hogwarts in *Harry Potter and the Sorcerer's Stone*).

Exercise: Reflect on your own call to adventure (how it happened), paying attention to your inner voice, chance encounters, a lecture you heard that prompted the call, a book you read, a feeling, a hunch or hint, someone saying 'you need to get your act together, this can't go on', your conscience. Notice the no and yes voices that urged/are urging the call to adventure (or getting help). How are you feeling/did you feel? Ambivalent? Excited? Reticent? Resentful?

Refusal of the Call

Although the Hero might be eager to accept the call (or not), at this stage he will have doubts, fears, hesitations. He will refuse the call and may suffer somehow as a result ('No, I don't need rehab/therapy, I'm fine'). The hardships he has to face may seem too much and the comfort of his home (inside his 'cave'/pub) may seem far more appealing to him than the perilous and unknown road outside. (e.g., Luke Skywalker tells Obi-Wan Kenobi that he can't go to Alderaan in *Star Wars*).

Exercise: What were your fears? What seemed too hard? Reflect on your leave-taking. Was it mental or physical? What were/are your contingency plans in case the adventure goes awry?

Meeting with the Mentor

At this crucial 'turning point', when the Hero really needs help and guidance (a 'hint from Heaven'), he meets a mentor figure (the archetype of the senex or Self), a guru or guide, who gives him something he requires – it could be advice, training, or self-confidence (a doctor, therapist, friend, family member). Whatever it is, it dispels his doubts and fears and gives him the strength of spirit required and the courage to begin his quest (e.g., Daniel LaRusso meets with Mr. Miyagi in *The Karate Kid*). The mentor may travel some way with the Hero or offer advice, and he/it may be human or even animal.

Exercise: Who or what helped you, if anybody? Who do you regard as a role model or mentor figure? Why? What are some of the challenges as you set off on your journey? What are your questions for the Guide? Formulate some. Be open to receiving a gift from the Guide (a mantra or talisman) to get you through later trials and tribulations. What guides might you need (wise mentoring)?

Crossing the Threshold

The Hero is ready to act upon his call to adventure and begin his quest (be it physical or spiritual). He may be pushed or pulled, driven, or drawn, but either way, he eventually goes voluntarily and crosses the threshold between the familiar (world) and the foreign (unfamiliar one). He may be attending an inpatient or outpatient clinic. We need to confront our inner demons. Myth can be looked at literally or symbolically (e.g., 'she's a dragon' or 'the demon drink'). The question is: What's keeping you stuck, and who or what is pulling you down?

Exercise: Here you can do a SWOT analysis. What are your heroic *strengths*? What are your *weaknesses*? What are your *obstacles*? What are your *threats* (such as dragons that need slaying; old haunts/pubs that still attract)? We need to re-introject our projections, integrate our shadow. If the 'home ground' is the tried and tested way, the call to adventure is a breakthrough (breakdown perhaps first) into the new/unfamiliar.

Tests, Allies, Enemies

Out of his comfort zone, the Hero is confronted with a series of challenges (initiations) that test him in a variety of ways. Obstacles cross his path which he must overcome. They could be physical hurdles or people intent on thwarting his designs. He needs to find out whom he can trust and whom he can't. He may meet allies but also enemies ('sure you don't have a problem'). Greater ordeals are yet to come. His skills are tested here, and the obstacles help him reach greater insight into his character and identity (e.g., Frodo leaves Rivendell with the Fellowship of the Ring and must learn how to be on the road as he travels in *The Lord of the Rings*).

Exercise: What obstacles have you overcome to be where you are now? What skill set do you still need? Whom do you trust? What insight(s) did you achieve? Who revealed themselves to be your friend or your 'enemy'? ('The enemy is the ego'.) List three exciting adventures or undertakings you have experienced – people, places, events, experiences, activities. What 'frogs' did you have to kiss? (How did you deal with rejections, hurdles?) What has stretched you, made you grow (perils and pitfalls)? What challenges have confounded you or made you stronger? What did you discover about yourself?

Approaching the Inner Cave: The Reward

The inmost cave may symbolise many things in the Hero's story such as an actual location in which lies a terrible danger or an inner conflict which the Hero hadn't to face up until now. Here he may once again face his fears and confront his doubts. He may need time to reflect on his journey so far – on the treacherous road he has taken in order to find the courage to continue. This brief respite helps the audience to appreciate and understand the magnitude of the ordeal that awaits him and escalates the tension in anticipation of his ultimate test. It can feel like everything's falling apart (e.g., Nero and Trinity gather an arsenal before heading off to rescue Morpheus in *The Matrix*).

Exercise: What have been your worries and insecurities, fears, and forebodings? Have you taken time out to see the big picture? Cite an instance when meaning has come from suffering. Give an example when you mobilised the 'defiant power of the human spirit'. Here we witness a confirmation or consolidation – a completion. It's all finally coming together. For example, an aha moment – the Archimedes' effect. What has yours been? It's like seizing the fire of the gods (e.g., Prometheus) or the sword (Arthur) or finding the Grail. Lessons here: patience, perseverance, preparation; letting go of ego; change in mindset (like peeling back layers of an onion); seeing differently.

Ordeal: Refusal of the Return

The supreme ordeal may be a dangerous physical test or a deep inner crisis the Hero (you) must face/confront in order to survive. It could be facing his greatest fear/phobia or most deadly foe. The Hero must draw on all his experiences and skills garnished and gathered thus far on the path to the inmost cave to overcome this challenge. Only through some form of 'death' can the Hero be reborn (a symbolic resurrection) that somehow grants him greater power or insight into his condition necessary to journey on and fulfil his destiny. This is the high point of his story where everything he holds dear is put on the line. If he fails, he dies, or life as he knows it will never be the same again (e.g., Dorothy and her friends battle the Wicked Witch in her castle in *The Wizard of Oz*).

Exercise: What would you say have been your three greatest challenges? How did you navigate your way through them? With this new encounter, it is hard to return/go back home (like the escaped prisoners in Plato's cave). The return can be as tough as the withdrawal (stages one to seven). So, what actions are you going to take to keep alive what you've learned? The reward needs protecting, e.g., lifelong learning, continuing professional support, ongoing therapy. A suggestion: read Homer's *Odyssey* (a Bible for homecoming heroes).

Reward: Seizing the Sword

After defeating 'the enemy', surviving 'death' and overcoming his greatest fear/ challenge, the Hero is transformed into a new state. He emerges from 'battle' (where he has slain his inner demons/dragons, addictions) a stronger, wiser person, often with a prize of some sort. This could be a new power or greater knowledge or wisdom or insight or even a reconciliation with a loved one or ally (reconciliation and recovery take the place of resentment). It will facilitate his return to the ordinary world (e.g., after the death of the dragon Smaug, Bilbo and the dwarves are free to help themselves to his treasure in *The Hobbit*).

Exercise: What did you have to overcome? What made you wiser? What did you gain or get from the experience? How do you hope to hang on to it?

The Return Road/Journey

The road back represents a reverse echo of the call to adventure in which the Hero had to cross the first threshold. Now he must return home with his reward, but this time the anticipation of danger is replaced with that of acclaim, vindication, absolution, exaltation, exoneration ('I'm so proud of you, son'). But still, the Hero's Journey is not yet over. He may still need one last push back into the ordinary world. He must choose between his own personal objective and that of a higher (impersonal/archetypal) cause or call (messianic mission; e.g., after the One Ring is destroyed, Frodo has a difficult time adapting to life as a normal hobbit in the Shire in *Return of the King*). Perhaps our Hero will now mentor others struggling with addiction and train to work as an addiction counsellor.

Exercise: Give an example of a conflict you experienced between a personal desire and an impersonal duty. You may be 'killed' on the return home. A prophet is never welcome in his own country – people will knock you down. You could be met with resentment, rage, envy, jealousy, especially from former friends. Your gift or grail could be resisted or rejected, critiqued, or condemned. Are you prepared for this? Not everyone will be pleased to see you safe and well. The wise Hero waits it all out. What or who has knocked you down? What roadblocks/traumas have you met along the way? How did you deal with them?

Resurrection

Apotheosis: This is the climax in which the Hero must face his final and most dangerous encounter with 'death'. This final battle represents something far greater than the Hero's own existence and its outcome, having far-reaching consequences for his ordinary world. If he fails, others will suffer (family members and friends, all too frequently), and this places more weight on his shoulders. We share in our Hero's hopes and trepidations. Ultimately, the Hero will succeed, destroy his 'enemy', and emerge from the battle reborn (e.g., the narrator must kill himself to stop Tyler Durden in *Fight Club*).

Exercise: Have you ever put your life on the line for anyone/anything? Or stuck your neck out (the giraffe principle)? What do you plan to do now? How will you live? What has replaced your now former addiction? If you're tempted again, to whom will you turn? Resurrection is seldom a once-off event.

Return with the Elixir

This is the final stage of the Hero's Journey when he returns home to his ordinary world a changed person. He will have grown, matured, learned many things, faced terrible dangers, but now looks forward to the start of a new life – addiction-free, for now, forever. His return brings fresh hope to those he left behind, or a solution to a problem, or a new perspective. His final reward could be a celebration or a Self-realisation. It represents three things: change, success, and proof of his journey. The Hero may return from whence he came, but things will never be the same again. For example, Luke, now a Jedi, restores balance to the Force and helps to bring peace to the galaxy; concurrently, he resolves his relationship with his father and is able to move on. There may be loneliness, but it is the opposite of lacklustre lethargy. Resolve assumes form in our post-addiction Hero's life.

Exercise: How have you grown? What life lessons have you learned? What does the future hold? What are you most looking forward to? Do more journeys await? Or is your role now to guide others? Or rest? Or become 'King'? What might that look like?

Apply the Hero's Journey to yourself. It is the perfect lens through which to view any change in your life. Plot your story of the hero. Write up 'My Hero's Journey' in a journal.

Summary Exercise: Twelve Reflective Questions to Consider

1   What was best and worst about your ordinary world? Give a brief biographical sketch of the ideas, events, and people who have been the greatest influence on your character.
2   What calls of adventure have you received and how did you respond to them? Have you ever had to deliver a call to adventure to anyone? What are you being called to do? When did you do something difficult or dangerous?
3   Have you ever refused a call, said no, hesitated? What were the consequences? In retrospect, were you right to have refused it or do you wish you had responded differently? What stopped you? Fear? Have you accepted anything that you wish you had refused?
4   What mentors have you most admired? What have they taught you? Have you helped/mentored anyone? Would you like to?

5 What have been the thresholds in your life that you had to cross? What have these times of transition, crossing, and change signalled for you? Did you have to give up anything?

6 Have you been tested in life? How? In what ways? By whom? Who has been an ally to you and who has been a foe/enemy?

7 Does conflict build you up or bring you down? What preparations do you make in advance of going 'into the cave', into 'the belly of the whale'? Do you ever want to go back? What demons or dragons have you encountered in the depths (internal or external challenges)? Is there a 'cave' (a contained space) where you would like to go?

8 Name some of the ordeals you have had to face. Did the suffering they entail make you stronger or teach you anything? How do you manage conflictual situations?

9 What rewards have you received in life? What recognitions? How did they make you feel?

10 What knowledge or wisdom or insight did you gain from times of crisis, from defeat or danger (risk)?

11 What character flaws do you still think you have? Which ones need to be corrected or worked on? What aspect of you got 'resurrected'? When do you feel most alive? What life lessons have you learned thus far?

12 What is your particular (personal) precious elixir? Do you keep it or share it? What use do you make of your talents? Where are they best deployed? How does your light shine? What do you think your legacy will be? What heals and helps you, providing you with happiness? What hinders that from happening?

Reflective Summary

Were there any surprises or disappointments on your Hero's Journey here? Who's the real hero in your life? Are you anyone's hero? Is your story worth telling? Where are you right now in your journey with addiction, would you say?

In James Joyce's *Ulysses* (the Latin name for Odysseus), there is more spiralling in the journey than straight lines (a process of fluidity rather than fixture – creative chaos). Its seventeen chapters last twenty-four hours on 16 June 1906. The book represents seventeen different lenses/ways to look at oneself. So, your journey may not be straight or straightforward. What matters is that you're moving, armed with a map and a heroic mindset. The path of the Hero, despite all its perils, is a path of promise, where all things are possible.

Chapter 8

Methods of Meditation

Lectio Divina

Both work in recovery (for example, the Twelve Steps of Alcoholics Anonymous [A.A.]) and the inner work of the Enneagram suggest daily meditation as the practice of presence to Self, a point I have been emphasising. In the Christian tradition, there is a monastic tradition known as *Lectio Divina*. A.A.'s fourth and twelfth steps will become the first step in contemplative meditation, so before we return to Thomas Keating and John Main (this time by explicating their methods of meditation), let us take a brief look at *Lectio Divina*.

Just as the subject is a threefold unity (body, soul, and spirit), there are three senses of Scripture – literal, moral, and spiritual. The Bible is a book that requires interpretation. *Lectio Divina* (divine reading) is an ancient Benedictine practice of reading passages from Scripture meditatively. Scripture is a sacrament and a *signum* – sign. We approach it with a listening heart. There are four levels of this spiritual practice (see Enzo Bianchi, *Lectio Divina*):

- *Lectio*: historical and literary level of the text – a loving and listening reading.
- *Meditatio*: the revelatory dimension – deeper meanings of the text emerge.
- *Oratio*: a dialogue with the divine ensues – silent prayer.
- *Contemplatio*: the search in Scripture for the face of God – divine indwelling.

Lectio invites us to ruminate on the Word in the following four ways, which I call the Four Rs.

- Read (*lectio*): reading the passage from Scripture attentively, asking 'What is it saying to me?'
- Reflect (*meditatio*): seeking to gain understanding of the passage, asking, 'How does the story relate to my situation?' as we peruse and pause over certain phrases to mull them over. We reflect on the meaning of God's Word.

DOI: 10.4324/9781003422570-9

- Respond (*oratio*): prayer, praise as one converses/communes with the Absolute/Almighty. We respond affectively through acts of devotion.
- Rest (*contemplatio*): abiding in the awareness of Presence. We rest in divine love.

Thomas Keating and Centering Prayer

The four guidelines for Centering Prayer are:

1 Choose a sacred word or sound (mantra in other traditions) as a symbol of your intention (consent) to the presence and action of the Absolute within you.
2 Sitting comfortably with eyes closed, settle and silently introduce the word to your practice.
3 Whenever thoughts (bodily sensations, feelings, images, etc.) engage you, return gently to the word.
4 At the end of the session, remain in silence with your eyes closed for a couple of minutes (see Keating, *Invitation to Love*, p. 16).

In *Open Mind, Open Heart*, Thomas Keating explores the practice of Centering Prayer, which begins from point four of *Lectio Divina* – resting in the Absolute. We thus:

- Consent to the presence of the Absolute.
- Surrender to the will of the Absolute.
- Relate to the Absolute in the cell of our heart, 'which is the silence of self'.

(Keating, *Open Mind, Open Heart*, p. 3)

The practice is commended by *Psalms* 46: 10: 'Be still and know that I am God'. This spiritual contemplative tradition was handed down by the Hesychasts of the Eastern Orthodox tradition and in particular by Pseudo-Dionysius (the sixth-century Syrian monk), Meister Eckhart, the Rhineland mystics of the Middle Ages, and the anonymous author of *The Cloud of Unknowing* in the fourteenth century, and later exemplified by the Carmelite tradition (Teresa of Avila, John of the Cross, Thérèse of Lisieux, and Elizabeth of the Trinity) and in the twentieth century by Thomas Merton.

Like the Enneagram, Centering Prayer elicits a commitment to the goal of transformation which takes place in the 'inner room' with a disposition of alert receptivity. It will involve the detachment from thoughts rather than their absence. A 'thought' is understood as any perception that appears on the inner screen of consciousness (a concept, a reflection, a body sensation, emotion, image, memory, noise, feeling). Centering Prayer is the art and act of attentiveness to a luminous Presence. One of the first effects of this spiritual practice is, according to Keating (Keating, *Open Mind, Open Heart*, p. 14), the release of the energies of the unconscious. Detachment is the goal, understood as a non-possessive, open attitude toward reality, a disposition that strikes at the root of the false self which is a 'monumental illusion' (Keating, *Open Mind, Open Heart*, p. 15). It's not just about attention but intention (consent). One intends to go into one's inmost being to encounter the divine indwelling. One says a sacred word which doesn't need to be repeated, but it does accompany one throughout the meditation. One's attention, indeed, is not even directed to the sacred word (syllable) or the mantra (in the John Main tradition). The word is a focal point, a placeholder. What separates us from the Absolute is the thought that we are separated, so thoughts are surrendered, let go of, dropped. Centering Prayer facilitates the process of inner transformation. One can be aware of thoughts but not engaged with thoughts. It's the thinking about thoughts that is problematic. The sacred word is a gesture, a symbol of one's consent (intention). Really, the sacred word is interior silence. The method of Centering Prayer is receptive rather than concentrative. The practice enables one to move into pure consciousness. As Keating observes: 'the place to which we are going is one in which the knower, the knowing, and that which is known are all one. Awareness alone remains. This is what divine union is' (Keating, *Open Mind, Open Heart*, p. 69). It's an exercise in letting go, either by ignoring thoughts or returning to the sacred word, as well as a process of liberation. Keating refers to the dynamism involved as a 'divine psychotherapy' (Keating, *Open Mind, Open Heart*, p. 95), in that the unconscious gets purified. Emotional experiences are stored in our bodies. With interior silence and resting in the Absolute, these emotional blocks begin to soften up. The emotional residue in our unconscious emerges in prayer. One simply releases them. One's natural resources of psychic health begin to be revived. Contemplative prayer brings about a change in our perception, one which involves 'a structural change of consciousness' (Keating, *Open Mind, Open Heart*, p. 97). Psychic wounds get healed through the 'unloading of the unconscious' (Keating, *Open Mind, Open Heart*, p. 98) and the work of God on the spiritual level of one's being (passive purification), as we get more in touch with our true Self. One accepts whatever comes down the stream of consciousness by cultivating a neutral attitude toward the psychological content of one's meditation. The meditation practice loosens all the rubbish, in Keating's analogy: 'It's like throwing out the garbage. You don't separate the eggshells from the orange peels. You just throw the whole thing out. Nobody is asking you to look through it or evaluate it' (Keating, *Open Mind, Open Heart*, p. 100). The purpose of Centering Prayer, Keating contends, is not to experience peace 'but to evacuate the unconscious obstacles to the permanent abiding state of union with God' (Keating, *Open Mind, Open Heart*, p. 102). The contemplative state is the aim, not contemplative prayer; not experiences but abiding awareness through 'the mysterious restructuring of consciousness' (Keating, *Open Mind, Open Heart*, p. 102). The 'false-self system' becomes dismantled. Letting go of (which is the principal discipline of Centering Prayer), incidentally, means not paying attention to. This requires opening to the Absolute 'at the level of the unconscious' (Keating, *Open Mind, Open Heart*, p. 103). Keating spells out the procedure thus: 'Do not resist any thoughts, do not retain any thoughts, do not react emotionally to any thought, and when you are engaged in some thought, return, ever so gently to the sacred word' (Keating, *Open Mind, Open Heart*, p. 104). In the interior silence, the Spirit (Self) heals our deepest wounds. Imagine the rays of the sun in a pool of water. The sun's rays are united to the water but distinct from it. The unconscious is purified by divine love in the contemplative process of transformation, and reality becomes more transparent in the process. 'Its divine Source will shine through it' (Keating, *Open Mind, Open Heart*, p. 107). Over time, everything in the unconscious will empty out (the process of purification) and the awareness of union with the Absolute will be continuous. Keating calls this 'the transforming union' (Keating, *Open Mind, Open Heart*, pp. 111–112). Centering prayer brings one to contemplative prayer, which is the prayer of quiet.

Keating distinguishes five types of thoughts (Keating, *Open Mind, Open Heart*, pp. 122–128):

- The wandering of the imagination (superficial thoughts that the imagination grinds out).
- Thoughts with an emotional attraction to them (when you get interested in something that's going on).
- Insights and psychological breakthroughs (our minds go on a fishing expedition, and we seem to have wonderful insights and breakthroughs).
- Self-reflection (a desire to reflect on what's happening may arise).
- Interior purification (the dynamic of divine psychotherapy).

Throughout this process, the undigested psychological material of a lifetime is gradually evacuated and the 'emotional investment of early childhood in programs for happiness based on instinctual drives is dismantled' (Keating, *Open Mind, Open Heart*, p. 126). It's important not to repress these thoughts but to let them pass through our awareness, accepting and letting them go. We thus:

- Resist no thought.
- Retain no thought.
- React emotionally to no thought.
- Return to the sacred word.

The sacred word is introduced inwardly 'as gently as laying a feather on a piece of absorbent cotton' (Keating, *Open Mind, Open Heart*, p. 178). Prayer is interior silence – the opening of body, mind, and heart to the Absolute. It's coming home to permeating Presence, which is at once both an emptiness and a fullness. It's not designed to bring one to a 'high' nor is it self-hypnosis. Keating concludes his book by highlighting our essential goodness, that the central aim is deification; that our true Self's centre of gravity is God; that 'God and our true Self are not separate. Though we are not God, God and our true Self are the same thing' (Keating, *Open Mind, Open Heart*, p. 158); that the false self develops in opposition to the true Self; that prolonged, pervasive, and paralysing guilt feelings come from the false self; that grace is in operation at every level and at every moment; that the journey to our true Self is the way to divine love; and that patience is hope in action.

Keating recommends meditating twice daily – once in the morning and once in the early evening – for twenty to thirty minutes. One might begin with a brief reading or relaxation exercise. At other times during the day, one can have recourse to what Keating calls an Active Prayer Sentence, such as 'O God, come to my aid, O Lord make haste to help me' (Cassian's formula), which, through repetition, gradually works its way into our subconscious memory. We remember that God's first language is silence (see Keating, *Open Mind, Open Heart*, p. 179).

The emotional programmes for happiness start as needs, grow into demands, then come 'shoulds'. Reality is expected to conform to my wishes. But, as Keating reminds us, 'repent' means '*to change the direction in which you are looking for happiness*' (Keating, *Invitation to Love*, pp. 11–12), which is a hangover from childhood. We pass through four levels of consciousness as we age, Keating maintains (Keating, *Invitation to Love*, pp. 31–37), following the work of Ken Wilber:

- Reptilian (0 to 2 years) – the day-to-day survival of needs such as food and shelter.
- Typhonic (2 to 4 years) – part-human, part-animal; in other words, the gradual emergence from one's instincts/body-self dominated by the need for survival, nourishment, and reproduction.
- Mythic membership (4 to 8 years) – the invention of language, providing a sense of belonging in the community and the development of the social self (socialisation).
- Mental egoic (8 years to adulthood) – the emergence of reason, full reflective self-consciousness.

Keating outlines four consents:

- In childhood, we are asked to consent to the basic goodness of our nature.
- In early adolescence, we are asked to accept the full development of our being by activating our creative talents.
- In early adulthood, we are asked to accept the fact of our nonbeing and the diminution of self through illness, old age, and death.
- Now, we consent to be transformed in the school of divine love.

(Keating, *Invitation to Love*, pp. 52–57)

In the transforming union, the dominance of the emotions ceases; former addictions and unhealthy attachments are replaced by newer connections and subtler energies. That said, Centering Prayer 'is not a magic carpet to bliss, a spiritual happy hour, a respectable substitute for mind-changing drugs, self-hypnosis, or a trance state' (Keating, *Invitation to Love*, p. 132). Its basic elements are solitude, silence, and simplicity. The emotional programmes for happiness are deliberately dismantled. Keating gives this advice: when you notice an upsetting emotion recurring frequently, name it without analysing it, then identify the event that triggered the emotion. Say: 'I give up my desire to control; I give up my desire for approval and affection; I give up my desire for security' (Keating, *Invitation to Love*, p. 154). Guarding the heart (consciousness) consists of letting go of emotional disturbance as soon as it arises and before one starts to think of it. This is the method for dismantling the programmes for happiness and the false self.

The key is to let go of the swirling thoughts of the *manas* mind. Keating likens them to boats passing by on the surface of a river. The river is a metaphor for human consciousness. The stream of consciousness resembles a river flowing toward the sea. The surface of the river stands for that level of consciousness that we use to attend to daily life. Sense perceptions, reflections, memories, images, feelings, and commentaries flow along the surface of our awareness like boats on a river. This is the ordinary level of consciousness. The river stands for the spiritual level of consciousness. By practising Centering Prayer (as a method of meditation), the mind becomes less dominated by external events and our emotional reactions to them. Spiritual attentiveness awakens. The depth of the river stands for the true Self and the divine Presence, the source of our life energies. Thus, four levels of awareness (see Keating, *Intimacy with God*, pp. 24–30):

- Ordinary level of consciousness
- Spiritual level of consciousness
- True Self
- Divine Presence

They are more like three concentric circles moving in from ordinary to spiritual awareness, then to the true Self at the heart of which is the divine Presence. When one begins to meditate, a circular motion is instituted with four major moments (see Keating, *Intimacy with God*, pp. 43–47):

- The introduction of the sacred word.
- Resting in the silence (freedom from attachments).
- The unloading of the unconscious (referring to the experience of psychic nausea that occurs in the form of a bombardment of thoughts and feelings that surge into awareness).
- Evacuation of this primitive material (we put up with the turbulence and return to the sacred word).

Centering Prayer, for Keating, is like going to a bad movie. We don't identify with the actors. We know we are in the cinema and can leave at any time. At the level of spiritual awareness, we are just witnessing what is going on in our lives (on screen) and are not captive to the plot (see Keating, *Intimacy with God*, p. 49). The Source lies in our inmost centre but is buried under the emotional debris of a lifetime. The motion in question is less circular and more resembling a spiral staircase to the Self. The divine archaeologist is at work, level by level. Centering prayer is consent to inner transformation. 'The false self is a master of delusion' (Keating, *Intimacy with God*, p. 72). But slowly our attachments are renounced and transformed. The higher the frequency (the more attuned we are to the Self), the greater the divine transmission. Abiding in deep peace *is* the method, while the source of Centering Prayer is the Trinity (*sat-chit-ananda*, or in Christian terms, God the Father, God the Son, God the Holy Spirit).

The Work of Cynthia Bourgeault

Cynthia Bourgeault, who closely follows (the late) Thomas Keating, makes the point that *Lectio Divina* is a necessary companion to Centering Prayer (see Bourgeault, *Centering Prayer and Inner Awakening*, p. vii) and that the inner observer is the bridge from interior silence to the blooming of the true Self. Centering Prayer is the art of awakening. Here, the advice in relation to the kenotic act of ego-emptying is '*If you catch yourself thinking, you let the thought go*' (Bourgeault, *Centering Prayer and Inner Awakening*, p. 23). The aim is not to stop the thoughts but to develop a detached attitude toward them. Meditation permits an interior rearrangement to go on. All the spiritual traditions share this same conviction: that humanity is the victim of a tragic case of mistaken identity – the confusion of the small/false self with the true Self. The false self is the ego (the unobserved mind,) while the true Self is the witness (Being Itself). The movement is from healing (psychotherapy) to holiness. This inner work involves paying less attention to the *contents* of consciousness (thoughts, feelings, reactions, desires, attractions, objects of addiction, etc.) and more attention to the *field* of consciousness (to the boats floating down the river, and the river itself). One shifts one's centre of gravity from the egoic orbit to Self-awareness. This deeper place 'watches *through* you' (Bourgeault, *Centering Prayer and Inner Awakening*, p. 127): presence without prejudice. What occurs during the discipline of Centering Prayer (and any practice of centering prayer associated with other spiritual traditions) is a rewiring of consciousness. Bourgeault calls it 'an upgrade in the operating system' (Bourgeault, *The Heart of Centering Prayer*, p. 5). She explains: 'Basically, the essence of the nondual consciousness is a quantitative change not in the object of perception but in the mechanics of perception' (Bourgeault, *The Heart of Centering Prayer*, p. 5). One begins to see from wholeness (nonseparation): holographic resonance – objectless awareness. The determining factor is the configuration of one's attention, not the content of the thought (as in cognitive therapy). Rumi, whom Bourgeault cites, employs the metaphor 'quivering like a drop of mercury' (Bourgeault, *The Heart of Centering Prayer*, p. 31) for this rewiring of consciousness. Centering Prayer is, thus, a witnessing practice. We pay attention not to *what* we are but to *that* we are. Thatness is being, whatness is being *that* (i.e., identification). Nonduality is the union that differentiates. Western 'contemplation' functions as the equivalent of nondual consciousness in the East. 'It is not a state of undifferentiated emptiness, but rather a state of profound, luminous awareness in which the individual components are suffused and drawn together by a single radiant Oneness like light pouring through a stained-glass window' (Bourgeault, *The Heart of Centering Prayer*, p. 167).

John Main's Christian Meditation

The Christian Meditation method of John Main, OSB, must also be mentioned. It was influenced by Eastern Advaita and, like Centering Prayer, seeks to dissolve all dualisms and dividedness. Similar advice to Keating's group – Contemplative Outreach – is given by the World Community of Christian Meditation (the work of John Main and Laurence Freeman, OSB):

1   Sit down and sit still with your back straight. Close your eyes lightly.
2   Interiorly, begin to recite a single word or mantra (such as 'Maranatha'; say it as four equal syllables).
3   Breathe normally, giving your full attention to the word as you say it, silently, gently, faithfully, and simply.

The difference is that Main advises that the mantra be repeated continuously (and also for twenty to thirty minutes twice daily). One sits still and in silence and begins to say a single word interiorly. Main recommends the word 'Maranatha' to be recited as four syllables of equal length. If images and thoughts come, return simply to saying the word (see Main, 'How to Meditate', *Word into Silence*, p. xvii). For Main, meditation is a process of learning to pay attention, to attend. One turns aside from what is passing to what is lasting, from the contingent to the necessary. The stillness of meditation is not passivity; rather, it is absorption, openness, full wakefulness. A thousand years after John Cassian (ca. AD 360–ca. AD 435), the anonymous author of *The Cloud of Unknowing* recommends the repetition of 'a little word' (chapter 39). The name for this prayer word is a *formula* in Latin, and in the Eastern tradition is known as a *mantra*. In meditation, the mind is restricted to the poverty of a single word/verse. The mantra is said in the mind (mental modality) at the beginning, but as we progress the mantra starts to sound not so much in our head as in our heart. As the *Maitri Upanishad* advises: the mind must be put in the heart. The mantra is like a harmonic that is sounded in the depths of one's spirit, deepening and bringing us to wholeness. The mantra is the device that does the work of meditation. Saying the mantra polishes the mirror within and enables us to find our true Self – the *Ātman* 'which is the means of becoming aware of union with the ultimate universal self, which is Brahman, which is God' (Main, *Word into Silence*, p. 19). The mantra is the key that opens the door to the secret chamber of the heart. Three stages are involved (see Main, *Word into Silence*, p. 20):

• Saying the mantra.
• Sounding the mantra.
• Listening to the mantra.

Through participation, we enter the still point. 'In meditation we must have the courage to attend solely to the Absolute' (Main, *Word into Silence*, p. 28). We may be bruised by surface distractions and subconscious anxiety, but at the deeper point, we progress through spheres of silence, ever deeper centres of being. The discursive operation of the intellect is set aside. Main observes: 'The mantra stills the mind and summons all our faculties to the resolution of a single point' (Main, *Word into Silence*, p. 41). It leads to integral awareness of the nature of our own being by bringing our mind centrewards. 'The way to silence is the way of the mantra' (Main, *Word into Silence*, p. 50). What it isn't is a spiritual anaesthesia. Main describes the mantra as 'the sacrament of our poverty in prayer' (Main, *Word into Silence*, p. 60). It brings us to the centre of our being, re-establishes conscious contact with the centre of all. 'The mantra leads us straight to this centre' (Main, *Word into Silence*, p. 65). The mantra is the sacrament of the present moment, one might say. The mantra guides us into deeper consciousness. It is the way of liberation. When the body is still, and the breath (*prāna*) is still, then the mind (*manas*) will come to stillness. When all three are still, one will be able to do the *dhyāna* (meditation). Meditation means remaining in the centre. The higher we toil up the mountainside, to deploy Main's analogy, the fainter becomes the mantra sounding in the valley below us. There will come a time when we enter the cloud of unknowing in which there is (absolute) silence 'and we can no longer hear the mantra' (Main, *The Inner Christ*, p. 67; also see Costello, *Between Speech and Silence: From Communicating to Meditating*). Such is the silence of the Absolute.

Chapter 9

Enneagram Applications

Introduction to the Enneagram

The Enneagram, approvingly cited by both Thomas Keating and Richard Rohr (indeed the latter has written several books on the topic), is a precise profiling instrument, a multidimensional model of consciousness that is complex, comprehensive, and complete. It is a nine-pointed symbol depicting nine different personality types. Each person has a dominant type that is dynamically connected to all other types. One can find out one's type by booking an Enneagram coaching session, reading the type descriptions, or doing an online assessment, for example, with Integrative Enneagram Solutions, which I suggest before proceeding. (The IEQ9 test is the most accurate on the market. It's an adaptive test that changes, through dynamic technology, the questionnaire items based on an individual's responses while also testing for mistyping. It measures the Enneagram profile, twenty-seven subtypes, centres, wings, lines, levels of integration, and six dimensions of stress and strain. It takes about thirty minutes to complete and is highly accurate with a validity rating of 95%.) I argue for the central usage of the Enneagram in any inner work. It is especially useful for addicted subjects, as it lays out the patterns of the ego-personality. It is an essential accompaniment to contemplative practice, journalling, and therapy.

The Enneagram shows our strengths and weaknesses, flaws, fixations, foundational fears, compulsions, blind spots, biases, and unconscious motivations as well as our potential for personal growth, development, change, integration, and core desires. It is uncannily accurate and extremely helpful in this regard for addicted subjects. The Enneagram reveals how our surface, shallow personality (functional ego) has stepped in to overshadow our essential nature (foundational Self), while pointing to a path out of the maze. It is a tool for transformation, one which integrates ancient spiritual insights with the contemporary psychology of personality, thus it is not only compatible with Advaita but fits it like a hand and glove. Only when we disidentify with ego can we reidentify with Self. The Enneagram describes what we're addicted to and how to become free from our fixations (see Costello, *The Nine Faces of Fear: Ego, Enneatype, Essence*).

DOI: 10.4324/9781003422570-10

The Nine Types

9 Adaptive Peacemaker
1 Strict Perfectionist
2 Considerate Helper
3 Competitive Achiever
4 Intense Creative
5 Quiet Specialist
6 Loyal Sceptic
7 Enthusiastic Visionary
8 Active Controller

Summary of the Types

Ones

Ones fixate on perfection; they focus on what's wrong. Theirs is a dualistic perception; they divide the world into perfect/imperfect, good/bad, right/wrong, black/white. Vulnerability is their core fear. Ones are principled, conscientious, structured, rigid, self-controlled, objectively discerning, and idealistic. Ones have a harsh inner critic. As with all the types, much will depend on the instincts, in other words, whether one has a social, sexual, or self-preservative subtype. 'There is only one way of doing things', Ones will say. They have a tendency to moralism. Their vulnerability is criticism; their value is goodness. Ones enact perfection. They are uptight in a mentally constructed morality rather than in essential conscience, as Almaas describes it (see Almaas, *Keys to the Enneagram*, p. 76). Self-Preservative Ones (SP1s) worry, plan a lot, are organised, find it hard to relax, engage in obsessive activities, have a heightened sense of what the ideal should be. They micromanage, are sticklers for details, and are tireless workers. Sexual Ones (SX1s) are intense, willing to express their anger, campaign for worthy causes, are pushy, impatient, wanting to improve things and people. They are energetic and reliable, can be charming, and have a high awareness of standards, but are stubborn and inflexible. They form intense relationships. Social Ones (SO1s) like to codify and guide others, love structure and procedures, and set high standards. They tend to keep their annoyance in check. They are calm, which often gives the impression of superiority. They are experienced as judgemental, uncompromising, and non-adaptable and can be excluded from groups on this account. They are convinced that they are right and want others to adapt to their viewpoint. Social Ones are self-sufficient and high-minded.

Twos

Twos are considerate helpers who can become resentful givers. They feel there is no love in the world and so they take care of everybody's needs. They are generous, available, adaptable, good listeners, fond of flattery, seductive, and ambitious, but they are not skilled in being explicit about what they want. They create a cycle of dependency. Their core fear is being unloved. Twos are sacrificing, people-centred, praising, friendly, concerned, warm-hearted, interactive. 'I love to love'. If their vulnerability is being unloved, their value is love. 'Merging love' is how Almaas describes the Helper Two (Almaas, *Keys to the Enneagram*, p. 55). Twos manipulate and flatter to get what they want from the idealised other. Hidden strings are attached to the Two's giving. The Two's overriding interest is investing in relationships, the more intense the better. They nourish because they need nourishment. Their inner emptiness is often converted into hysterical symptoms. Self-Preservative Twos (SP2s) are self-nurturing, but behind this veneer of selfless giving is the strong need for approval. They are competent and guarded, ambivalent about their relationships, and slow to trust. They may resort to sulking if their needs are not met. Theirs is a 'giving-to-get' syndrome. They are sensitive and easily hurt. They are good planners and supportive. Sexual Twos (SX2s) believe life is about inspiring passion in others. They are frequently detached from their own needs, so intent are they on creating powerful connections with others. They weave all sorts of people together and win them over. They are helper-givers. They are passionate and strong-willed but can become aggressive. They take on their partner's interests to create a perfect union and have difficulty letting go if things don't work out. Social Twos (SO2s) attract preferential treatment and work best when their talents are recognised and deployed. They like to present a powerful persona. Theirs is a strategic giving. They are sincere in helping others, but they can move more to the powerful and the prestigious, overlooking others in the process. They may exploit or manipulate unconsciously. They are big-picture people.

Threes

Threes are competitive achievers, ambitious, efficient, productive, driven, goal-oriented, busy, practical, focused. They have workaholic tendencies and love to outshine others. Their need is to be seen as successful and look good. They're shape-shifters, chameleons, duplicitous. They care about their image; they desire to be the best. They are good organisers and live life in the fast lane. 'I have to be 101 different people'; 'I change the message to suit the audience'; 'Every engagement is a war'. Their vulnerability is the fear of being worthless; their value is effectiveness. Self-Preservative Threes (SP3s) are single-minded and have a strong work ethic. They are independent and desire to be invaluable. They don't openly seek recognition, preferring that their work speaks for them. They may want to look successful, but they don't want others to know they want this, lest they be seen as superficial. They are ambitious and have the ability to overcome adversity. Their need to quell anxiety might lead to workaholism. They are not so in touch with their feelings. Others can perceive them as arrogant. They are very connected to image and interpret the world and others according to a measurement of success and achievement. They want to be the star, valued highly by society. They are the most extroverted of all the Enneatypes. They act as role models and paragons. Almaas has this to say about them: 'They might become famous – a movie or sports star – but they do not shine in their inner world. Their shine is worldly and fake' (Almaas, *Keys to the Enneagram*, p. 92). Sexual Threes (SX3s) are trusted cheerleaders. They focus on what is good for the family or group. They prefer to work to support others. They find it difficult to promote themselves. They tend to attract other talented people to the team. They take criticism personally. This triggers their fear of disappointing others. They want to be seen as the perfect partner. They experience an inner emptiness and can become disconnected from their emotions, though they may experience sporadic sadness. Social Threes (SO3s) are dynamic and lead with confidence. They are hardworking and humorous and make a good first impression. Prestige, admiration, and applause are important to them. They enjoy being the centre of attention. They are likely to lead in whatever capacity they find themselves. They desire social success and indeed are driven by it. They are adaptable and like to show off their homes, titles, clothes, cars, or jewellery. They work hard to create a pleasing image, discouraging overt familiarity.

Fours

Fours are intense creatives, sensitive, aesthetic (love of beauty), deep, emotional, expressive, individualistic, self-attuned, inspired, introspective, moody, dramatic, courageous, purpose-driven, tenacious. They are often the black sheep of the family. They can live in a fantasy world, full of longing. Many artists are Fours. 'I don't do superficiality', 'I hate small talk', 'I get depressed in visually ugly spaces', 'I'm sensitive to criticism', 'Melancholy gives me meaning', 'I don't do fake and boring', 'I'm intolerant of superficial happiness', 'I feel lonely and misunderstood', 'I'm set apart'. Their vulnerability (blind spot) is being ordinary, while their value is originality. Self-Preservative Fours (SP4s) are fearless, tenacious, resilient, and positive. Authenticity is important to them. They champion others, often to detach from their own pain. They want what others have. What they long for tends to be out of reach. Abundance eludes them. They suffer quietly and are strong in the face of pain, disguising their frustrations to avoid revealing envy or shame. They are sensitive but appear happy and steadfast. Slowing down causes them distress. Sometimes they self-sabotage and work against themselves. They avoid addressing deeper underlying problems. The Four is the tragic type with an aesthetic acumen. Van Gogh was probably a Four. They are missing something in themselves. They lack a stable identity. They need control (it steadies them). Sexual Fours (SX4s) are often impulsive and impatient and tend to be outspoken. They measure themselves against others, so that others may experience them as arrogant. As they tend not to acknowledge their envy, it can come out as anger.

They experience criticism as an attack. They are highly romantic in their pursuit of a partner, even if loving warmth does not come naturally to them. Their unexpected anger can confuse others. They are future- and action-oriented. Social Fours (SO4s) are emotionally aware and empathic, and can beat themselves up for being weak. They will experience a sense of inferiority. They tend to hide their feelings from others but can express them to those whom they love. They can dwell on things and engage in drama. They see their suffering as special and tend to define themselves via their emotions. They see themselves frequently as having come off second best. They have a deep-seated competitive side and want to be recognised.

Fives

Fives are quiet specialists, perceptive, curious, competent, conceptual, cerebral, detached, reflective, private, shy, unsentimental, self-sufficient, inventive, and innovative. Fives want to understand and make sense of the world. Their avarice is for knowledge. They are looking for ultimate meaning. They don't like being put on the spot or being made to feel dependent on anyone. Their vulnerability is about looking foolish. Their value is wisdom (knowledge is important to these thinking types). Fives love to analyse and solve problems, be experts in their domain. They avoid the interior life, self-isolate, compartmentalise, and detest improvisation. They can keep secrets, sometimes are provocateurs, and are avaricious for information. They feel that the world invades their privacy. 'Knowledge is never enough. I live in my head', 'I don't like last-minute surprises', 'I'm selfish with my time', 'I struggle to comfort others'. Self-Preservative Fives (SP5s) are inquisitive; intelligent; and eager to understand philosophy, religion, and science. They like boundaries and independence. They believe they have limited time, space, energy, and resources so these are allocated sparingly. Selective in whom they allow behind the walls of their fortress of solitude, they form small groups of trusted friends where their kindness and humour are appreciated. They tend to withdraw in silence rather than show anger, but they can be cutting when their vulnerabilities are triggered. They are quiet and reflective and lean towards the lone scholar. They can lead a frugal life. They shy away from receiving recognition and rely on the contributions of others. The primary defence of the Five is emotional avoidance and distancing. They are introverted investigators. They are cerebral knowers. Fives want enlightenment (probable examples: Freud and the Buddha). Fives love insight; their world is governed by objectivity and observation. Sexual Fives (SX5s) are creative, artistic, intense, romantic, sensitive, and attuned to the feelings of others. This countertype values human relationships and is passionate about finding that special person with whom they can feel safe. They highly prize trust and conduct themselves with transparency. They can be isolated from the external world. They set the bar high for significant others. They are committed to creativity. Social Fives (SO5s) are inclined to inquisitiveness.

They deeply investigate matters and uncover and synthesise them. They search for the essence or meaning of a situation and pursue wisdom. They connect with like-minded seekers. They are idealistic, and oversimplify things at times. They can idealise people based on their knowledge. They prioritise intellectual connections over emotional ones. They can appear arrogant, but they are like-able, amusing, and outgoing. They can seek out an expert, putting them on a pedestal. They secretly seek admiration.

Sixes

Sixes are loyal sceptics. They are devoted, prepared, trustworthy, team-oriented, suspicious, anxious, alert (indeed hypervigilant), and responsible. Their emotional state is angst. They are dutiful, unsure, feel pressure, anticipate the worst, possess an inferiority complex, are security conscious if not downright para-noiac, and phobic. They fear being unprepared and value loyalty above all else. Self-Preservative Sixes (SP6s) are warm diplomatic, generous, caring, affection-ate. They are sensitive, considerate, compassionate, fair, good communicators, and have a win–win attitude in negotiations. They can be unsure of themselves and hesitant, as well as cautious, but they build supportive alliances and accu-mulate relationships to assuage their anxiety, forging connections of exchange. Their home is their comfort/castle where they are shielded and secure. They seek out a protective partner and do their best not to disappoint. They hold back their aggression. They tend to be calm and action-oriented in crises. Sexual Sixes (SX6s) face fear and seek to protect themselves and others from possible dangers. Theirs is a powerful presence. They present themselves as bold and fearless. They don't tolerate weakness. They like to tackle things head-on. They are daredevils. They see the world as a threatening place. They do their utmost to avoid being taken advantage of. They adopt the contrarian response in de-bates and like to counter others in discussion. They hide behind a paranoid façade. The traits of the Six are stubbornness, hard-headedness, an 'unyielding determination, and a refusal to listen to listen to others' (Almaas, *Keys to the Enneagram*, p. 41). Hitler embodied the extreme, paranoid character of the Six. His personal will became a *libido dominandi*. Social Sixes (SO6s) are intelligent, strategic thinkers with a clear sense of duty. They enjoy being of service. They uphold law, order, and structures. They like diagrams and flowcharts. They tend to pessimism. Their approach can be rigid and inflexible. They are astute and insightful, meticulous and efficient, respectful, rule-based, and humble. They have difficulty trusting opinions but are impressed by authority figures.

Sevens

They are thinkers whose vice is gluttony – they always want more, and need to avoid pain, limitation, and any restrictions on their liberty at all costs. They are fearful (though this is rarely shown), hedonistic, epicurean, indulgent, excessive, and juggle things. They have monkey minds and find it hard to endure the present, getting bored easily and looking for endless distractions. They plan and anticipate, living in the future. They are adventurous, gourmets, *bon vivants*, social butterflies who always have a plan B. Sevens are dispersive, can be childlike, and are great synthesisers. They skim, live at a fast pace, and like the quick fix. 'I'm on a speed train', 'Is this going to take long?', 'I can't wait', 'What's next?' They tend to reframe and look at life through rose-coloured glasses; see the silver lining of every cloud; value joy, happiness, and positivity. They can be a lot to handle. Stress is paralysing for Sevens; they ignore what's stressing them and also turn away from the boredom of mundane tasks and issues. Sevens want existential freedom and novelty more than anything. John Luckovich (an Enneagram teacher) describes the gluttony of the Seven's passion as 'an inability to know what's going to satisfy them' (in his comments on December 9 at the annual Enneagram Global Summit, 2021). Sevens feel they didn't get what they needed in childhood, and though they can be very emotional, they are not grounded in their heart centre. They are not good at limiting their feelings or closing off possibilities. They hide their suffering, as they want to be a light in the world. For the Seven, satisfaction is always just around the corner. Theirs is a voracity for experience. They accelerate through life. For the Seven, pain is a place of no return. They are energisers with a buzz about them, but how much will be enough for the Seven? They are great integrators, exuberant, and exultant, but they are called to moderation. Unconsciously, they yearn to connect to essential freedom and sober joy. 'Pleasure vehicle' is how Almaas describes the world of the Seven (Almaas, *Keys to the Enneagram*, p. 107). Sevens are dilettantes, always planning for what they believe will bring them pleasure. They are perky, buoyant, and carefree but become bored when things become repetitive. They dislike being pinned down and shun suffering. They sample everything rather than settle for anything. An unliberated Seven might be a hedonist, but an awakened one is Sri Aurobindo. Spiritual awakening is the beyond of psychological liberation. Self-Preservative Sevens (SP7s) usually get what they want; are always alert to new possibilities; are friendly, playful, and talkative. They are reciprocally loyal to friends. They are self-referencing with their shadow side being selfishness. Their two main drives are an insatiable desire for pleasure and a preoccupation with getting what they need. They want the best for everyone, but they also ensure that they have what they need to have fun and feel secure. Having a wealth of resources (financial, personal, etc.) is important to them. Sensing a shortage in these can fill Sevens with fear. They are intelligent (seeking endless mental stimulation), calculating, and quick to capitalise on opportunities. Their social skills are finely tuned. They feel unrestricted by rules and are adept at developing rationalisations. They have a hunger to consume as many enjoyable experiences as possible and seek to escape life's unpleasantness and discomfort. They are practical, have a positive attitude, are entrepreneurial, and leverage their strengths and assets in business even if they leave a trail of unfinished projects behind them. Sexual Sevens (SX7s) are cheerful but impressionable. They tend to be idealistic and blind to pain. They see the world in a dreamy way; they escape pain through positivity and happiness. They fantasise about the world being a delightful place and so avoid the more daunting and darker aspects of human existence. They test limits through humour and seduction and seek approval and appreciation. They won't want to miss out on anything. They try to ensure life is a spectacular show. They are easily swayed, however, by others and can be quite gullible/impressionable, so much so that they embrace and adopt the ideas of others with alacrity. They're anxiously restless and can become passive–aggressive if things or people oppose them. In love, they desire a mystical connection, honouring communion. They intensely dislike being bored and are always pursuing the next thing. Social Sevens (SO7s; the countertype) are dutiful, zestful, and self-aware. They are forward-looking idealists who champion social change. They serve others (are sacrificing), often sacrificing their own needs in the process, avoiding excess (unlike other Sevens). Their philanthropy can conceal guilt for wanting either enjoyment or acting in self-interest. They are warm and expressive and channel their energy into creating a world free of conflict. They are generous and dedicated but can become exhausted and depleted. They look for the perfect partner.

Eights

Eights are active controllers, powerful, direct, dominant, decisive, determined, blunt, frank, power-oriented, and confrontational. They take charge and don't hold back. They avoid weakness and vulnerability, are a true force of nature. They make things happen but are overwhelming – their recipients can feel attacked/assaulted by them. They are intense, influential, self-assured, and protective. 'I need to win/prevail'. They are the boss, authoritative, excessive, courageous, controlling, active, motivated, assertive/aggressive, and piqued by injustices. They can be vengeful. 'They said I was a bully; I thought I was an angel', 'Tell me it can't be done, and I'll see it is done', 'I love opinions, but I'm usually right', 'I don't like chit chat', 'I continue until I crash hard'. Eights hate to be controlled. They can come across as intimidating. Deep down in an Eight there is a needy child. Self-Preservative Eights (SP8s) are strong and assume a mentor or paternal role. They are hardworking and have a flair for the deal, for trading and negotiating. They are selfish under strain but also generous and loyal. They are assertive in expression, and single-minded in pursuit of what they want. They are intolerant of incompetence. They can disregard the opinions of others. They are straightforward but can equally keep their cards close to their chest. They are forthright and can overlook feelings. They are enduringly self-reliant. Sexual Eights (SX8s) are passionate, intense, charismatic, and warm, and ensure they are the centre of attention. They can act impulsively and become iconoclasts and trailblazers. Material things don't particularly satisfy or interest them, but they do value power and attention. They can be demanding and are inclined to detach from their intellect. Unconsciously, they seek a true equal. They form close relationships and either become dominant in their relationships or make their partners dependent on them. They are natural-born leaders. Eights use belligerence as a way of being in the world – they are often boisterous and bullying. As Almaas describes it, theirs is the 'rage in the service of revenge' (Almaas, *Keys to the Enneagram*, p. 33). Social Eights (SO8s) focus on justice and society, becoming warriors in the service of change. They are cooperative and lead by example. They are good listeners and can take criticism; they forge close alliances. They are concerned about infringements and injustices, exploitation, and inequities. They can lose touch with their need for love in their desire to be protectors. They can lean towards overconfidence (cockiness) and self-absorption. Behind their supportive demeanour is a hidden fear of abandonment.

Nines

Nines are adaptive peacemakers, mediators, patient, supportive, genuine, affable, unassuming, easy-going, chilled, calm, laid back, accommodating, accepting, fair, withdrawn, indolent/slothful. They see all views. They are gut-centred and avoid conflict. Nines are stubborn as mules; they do what they want. They like to keep the balance and stick to their comfortable routines. They can become passive–aggressive when triggered. Theirs is a spiritual laziness – *acedia*. They feel they don't matter; they fade into the background and tend not to stand up for themselves. They're diplomatic, slow as a snail, obliging, have difficulty in affirming/asserting themselves, forget their own needs, can be couch potatoes, operate on cruise control, suffer from inertia, procrastinate, and have rare explosions/outbursts of rage. They self-soothe through narcotisation and numbing out – they go to sleep. 'I perceive life as a web of connections not as linear', 'I want to understand the big picture', 'I want peace to prevail and avoid conflict, both external and internal', 'It takes a lot of energy for me to find out my wants', 'I go along with the crowd', 'I'm OK if everybody else is OK'. Self-Preservative Nines (SP9s) are reliable and consistent. They appreciate the simple things of life, such as watching television, eating, and drinking. They put their physical needs first. They can lose their sense of time as well as themselves. Theirs is a straightforward life – they overlook their deeper needs. They prefer familiar routines to adventure. Peace and alone time are important for them, lest they become irritable and obdurate. They focus on immediate experiences and are a lot less interested in philosophical perspectives. They are private and have an ironic sense of humour. If they feel others are trying to control them, they do not budge from their position. Sexual Nines (SX9s) are receptive and non-judgemental, persevering, and tolerant. They seek the perfect partner with whom to bond. They blend with people, are gentle, and thoughtful, as well as loyal in love, but they are uncertain as to who they really are and so can adopt the viewpoints of those closest to them as they struggle to feel grounded or anchored in themselves. They live vicariously and virtually through others but become passive–aggressive when their own needs are not being met. They deny their individuality and struggle to find their purpose. They are indecisive and rely on cues and clues from others. They can find it difficult to connect with others. 'Boundless love' is how Almaas describes the world of the Nine (Almaas, *Keys to the Enneagram*, p. 123). Nines are asleep to what reality is and are unconscious of who they really are. Ego-indolence characterises this peacemaker. They are often narrow and literal, and despise conflict and confrontation. They opt for peace and comfort and the absence of challenge. Social Nines (SO9s) are lively and outspoken, fun-loving, and extroverted. They enjoy working with others. They are often the glue holding disparate groups together cohesively. They are impressive negotiators. They put their attention on being accepted by the group. They are servant-leaders. They find it hard to say no and work long and hard. They avoid connecting with their deepest self, however. Beneath their bonhomie and congeniality is a melancholy which stems from their deep-seated sense that they don't fit in. They are neutral and detached from their emotions.

These nine paths are portals to essence.

Nine Addictions

It's important to bear in mind that all nine Enneagram types can have any kind of addiction.

- Nines are addicted to keeping the peace, to self-forgetfulness, and to accommodating others. Their potential pathology is dissociative disorder. They might use marijuana or narcotics to deaden their feeling of loneliness and anxiety or mind-expanding substances in their desire to merge.
- Ones are addicted to perfection, order, worrying, and dwelling on their defects. Their potential pathology is obsessive–compulsive disorder. Their addictions will often be private and could include over- or undereating, anorexia, and bulimia.
- Twos are addicted to giving (in order to get), to being 'generous', and collecting needy people in order to control them. Their potential pathology is histrionic personality disorder. They may binge if feeling 'love-starved' and use substances as need replacements.
- Threes are addicted to achieving/accomplishing, being desired, and being their best in terms of performance. Their potential pathology is narcissistic personality disorder. They may become workaholics, and this could lead them to excessive intake of stimulants/amphetamines.
- Fours are addicted to the intensity of feeling; the siren call of fantasy seduces them. Their potential pathology is depression. They may take antidepressants to anaesthetise their melancholy or overindulge in eating for the purposes of emotional consolation.

- Fives are addicted to knowledge/information, to problem-solving and investigating, to isolating and withdrawing. Their potential pathology is schizoid personality disorder. They may develop poor eating and sleeping habits due to minimising their own needs and thus neglect nutrition, perhaps using psychotropic drugs for mental stimulation or to disappear.
- Sixes are addicted to doing their duty, to security and reassurance, to insurance. Their potential pathology is paranoid and/or borderline personality disorder. This type shows a greater susceptibility to alcoholism than many other types; they are prone to dependency of all kinds and may use amphetamines for stamina.
- Sevens are addicted to new experiences/pleasure and being free, to excess and escape, to future planning. 'Sevens are caught in a cycle of anticipation, craving, and excess that we call the chocolate syndrome' (Riso and Hudson, *The Wisdom of the Enneagram*, p. 279). Their potential pathology is manic–depressive disorder. This type is most prone to addictions. They will use stimulants (coffee, cocaine), painkillers, alcohol, narcotics, and psychotropics; have cosmetic surgery; and can get hooked on almost anything.
- Eights are addicted to control, taking charge, winning, and their own self-sufficiency ('If you want something done, you have to do it yourself'). Their potential pathology is antisocial personality disorder. They tend to avoid medical visits and ignore their physical needs, and so indulge in alcohol as a way of pushing themselves hard. They are susceptible to stress, strokes, and heart conditions. They can become adrenaline junkies.

The Core Motivations

9 Have to keep balance
1 Have to do the right thing
2 Have to be liked
3 Have to outshine the rest
4 Have to be unique
5 Have to understand
6 Have to be safe
7 Have to experience it all
8 Have to be in control

Defence Mechanisms

These are the defence mechanisms associated with each Enneagram type:

- Ones: reaction formation
- Twos: repression
- Threes: identification
- Fours: fantasy/introjection

- Fives: isolation
- Sixes: projection
- Sevens: rationalisation
- Eights: denial
- Nines: narcotisation

Personality Disorders

The personality disorders associated with each unredeemed Enneagram type are:

- Ones: obsessive–compulsive
- Twos: dependent
- Threes: narcissistic
- Fours: bipolar
- Fives: schizoid
- Sixes: paranoid
- Sevens: ADHD/melancholic
- Eights: sociopathic
- Nines: passive–aggressive

Nine Temperaments

These are the nine temperaments that researchers (see Thomas and Chess, *Temperament and Development*, 1977) found in babies that held true to adulthood (this study was independent of any knowledge of the Enneagram) alongside the correlated Enneagram types (per the work of Dr David Daniels):

- Ones: self-regulating
- Twos: socially contactful
- Threes: active
- Fours: socially sensitive
- Fives: socially held back
- Sixes: fearful
- Sevens: playful
- Eights: difficult/demanding
- Nines: compliant/easy

Spiritual transformation can happen in a flash, a flicker, or a flow. The Self is an innate guidance system. Above, we have a summary of the ego types. To know one's type is not to stereotype, but we are born with our type, which is unchanging over the course of our lives. The Enneagram (from *ennea* meaning 'nine' and *gram* meaning 'what is drawn') shows nine core motivations, archetypes. Its origin can be traced back to Plato, Plotinus (author of the *Enneads*), the Desert Fathers, and Sufi mystics, but in the twentieth century those most responsible for its use were G. I. Gurdjieff (1866–1949) in the 1920s, the Russian philosopher and spiritual teacher (founder of the Fourth Way); followed by Oscar Ichazo (1931–2020), the Bolivian philosopher (founder of the Arica Institute); and Claudio Naranjo (1932–2019), the Chilean psychiatrist in the 1970s, who was the principal developer of the Enneagram of Personality, continuing on with a host of others from the 1980s (when I discovered it) and beyond. Where other personality programmes show behaviour (outer), the Enneagram emphasises motivation (inner).

'Virtues' are expressions of our essence; 'Passions' point to our maladaptive habits. Unlike the ego types, the essential qualities are called 'Holy Ideas' (Divine Forms) in the Enneagram tradition. Each Holy Idea has a corresponding Virtue (an essential quality of the heart), which is experienced by us when we abide in essence. As we lose this awareness and fall away from essence into the trance of personality, these Holy Ideas become a person's ego fixations. And the loss of contact with Virtue causes the person's characteristic Passion. There are three centres of intelligence, which we all share: thinking, feeling, and instinct (gut). We can describe them thus:

- Head: dominant in types 5, 6, and 7
- Heart: dominant in types 2, 3, and 4
- Hands/action: dominant in types 8, 9, and 1

- What is to be done? – The action centre is hot and corresponds to the instinctual centre of the brain.
- How do I feel? – The feeling centre is warm and corresponds to the limbic system of the brain.
- What do I know? – The thinking centre is cool and corresponds to the prefrontal cortex of the brain.

Types	Emotional Issues	Centre
Eights, Nines, Ones	Anger, control	Body
Twos, Threes, Fours	Sadness, grief, self-esteem	Heart
Fives, Sixes, Sevens	Fear, anxiety	Head

These can stacked differently so one might think first, act second, and feel last. We all have one core type, but we also have secondary and tertiary types within each of the other two centres (fixation). These two 'fixes' combined with our core type produce our Trifix (for example, one might be a SP784, in other words, a Self-Preservative Seven with an Eight and Four). Trifix refers to centre-specific style – to what's most pronounced in the centre. This dominant type represents the ego's preferred defence strategy, and it will deploy the other two types to make decisions. The high side of the intersection of these three Enneagram types defines what gives life direction and purpose; the low side is that the defence strategies miss the mark, preventing a person from achieving a higher level of self-awareness. It is best if the three types work in concert with one another rather than collision. Each Trifix creates a type unto itself.

The Twenty-Seven Subtypes

Katherine Fauvre studied this topic in detail and provided the names associated with the twenty-seven Trifix archetypes, together with descriptions (see www. katherinefauvre.com; also Beatrice Chestnut, *The Complete Enneagram*):

- The Mentor (125, 152, 215, 251, 512, 521)
- The Supporter (126, 162, 216, 261, 612, 621)
- The Teacher (127, 172, 217, 712, 721)
- The Technical Expert (135, 153, 315, 513, 531)
- The Taskmaster (136, 163, 316, 361, 613, 631)
- The System Builder (137, 173, 317, 371, 713, 731)
- The Researcher (145, 154, 415, 451, 514, 541)
- The Philosopher (146, 164, 416, 461, 614, 641)
- The Visionary (147, 174, 417, 471, 714, 741)
- The Strategist (258, 285, 528, 582, 825, 852)
- The Problem Solver (259, 295, 529, 592, 925, 952)
- The Rescuer (268, 286, 628, 682, 826, 862)
- The Good Samaritan (269, 296, 629, 692, 926, 962)
- The Free Spirit (278, 287, 728, 782, 827, 872)
- The Peacemaker (279, 297, 729, 792, 927, 972)
- The Solution Master (358, 385, 538, 583, 835, 853)
- The Thinker (359, 395, 539, 593, 935, 953)
- The Justice Fighter (368, 386, 638, 683, 836, 863)
- The Mediator (369, 396, 639, 693, 936, 963)
- The Mover Shaker (378, 397, 738, 783, 837, 873)
- The Ambassador (379, 397, 739, 793, 937, 973)
- The Scholar (458, 485, 548, 584, 845, 854)
- The Contemplative (459, 495, 549, 594, 945, 954)
- The Truth-Teller (468, 486, 648, 684, 846, 864)
- The Seeker (469, 496, 649, 694, 946, 964)
- The Messenger (478, 487, 748, 784, 847, 874)
- The Gentle Spirit (479, 497, 749, 794, 947, 974)

Three Centres

When we're present to the centre (essence), then:

- The body is alive, relaxed, and grounded.
- The heart is open, connected, and receptive.
- The mind is calm, quiet, and still.

We can engage in yoga or Aikido or dance to help us become more mindful of our bodies, practice gratitude and compassion to ensure our hearts don't close, and read the words of the wise or the scriptures to ensure we're guarding what is entering our minds (of course, they all interconnect). The journey of integration (from unhealthy, through average, to healthy/redeemed) involves the movement from:

Vice (Passion) to Virtue:	Heart centre
Fixation (mental) to Holy Idea:	Head centre
Instincts to Awareness:	Gut centre

When the Holy Ideas become distorted this results in fixations in the head, passions in the heart, and instincts in the gut. By recalling the Virtue in a state of presence, the particular Passion can be transformed. The process is twofold:

• Restoration of the Virtue
• Transformation of the Passion

The Holy Ideas represent the nondual perspectives of essence (ways of knowing the unity of being). They are what naturally arise in a still mind – when we are (spiritually) awake. The loss of them leads to the ego's delusions about self and reality called the type's ego fixations/compulsions. Compulsions are the neurotic ways we respond to events – they are automatic reactions to the stresses and strains of life. They are autonomic repetitions of internal psychic strategies. Through the ego fixation, the person is trying to restore the balance/ freedom of the Holy Ideas, but from the dualistic point of view of the ego, which ultimately fails. The Holy Ideas function as antidotes to the ego fixations. Let's summarise the Enneagram of the Virtues, the Passions, the Ego Fixations, and the Holy Ideas next.

Enneagram of the Virtues

9 Right action
1 Serenity
2 Humility
3 Truthfulness
4 Equanimity
5 Non-attachment
6 Courage
7 Sobriety
8 Innocence

Each Enneagram type has a Virtue that balances its Vice. The Virtues refer to the strengths that flow from a more self-aware perspective on the world. They are positive behaviours that support the expression of our essential Self.

Enneagram of the Passions (Vices)

9 Sloth
1 Anger
2 Pride
3 Deceit
4 Envy
5 Avarice
6 Fear
7 Gluttony
8 Lust

Each Enneagram type has a Vice (or Passion) that flows from our subjective, distorted worldview. Vices are unhealthy habits and behaviours that give the impression they are helping us to manage our various challenges, but they are not authentic and function only in a limited way.

Enneagram of the Ego Fixations

9 Indolence
1 Resentment
2 Flattery
3 Vanity
4 Melancholy
5 Stinginess
6 Cowardice
7 Planning
8 Vengeance

Fixations are distorted ideas that drive the type's thinking, feeling, and action – the core coping patterns for that type. Fixations focus on who we should/are supposed to be. They are driven by our fears.

Enneagram of the Holy Ideas

9 Holy Love
1 Holy Perfection
2 Holy Will/Freedom
3 Holy Law/Hope
4 Holy Origin
5 Holy Omniscience/Transparency
6 Holy Faith
7 Holy Wisdom/Plan
8 Holy Truth

Holy Ideas are universal truths that help each type broaden their perspective if they can only connect to them. They are the antidote to each Enneagram type's Fixation, representing reality as it is when seen through unfiltered eyes. If the Passions are the nine ways whereby the heart gets stuck, the Virtues are the nine spiritual attitudes that counteract the Passions. The Holy Ideas are nine spiritually enlightened perspectives that underlie the personality Fixations. They are the faces of nondual realisation. As Almaas puts it in his *Keys to the Enneagram*, 'Such a liberation is a nondual realization of reality' (Almaas, *Keys to the Enneagram*, p. 7).

Summary

Type	Holy Idea	Virtue	Passion/Vice	Fixation
9	Love	Action	Slothfulness	Indolence/ Laziness
1	Perfection	Serenity	Anger	Resentment
2	Will/Freedom	Humility	Pride	Flattery
3	Hope	Truthfulness	Deceit	Vanity
4	Origin	Equanimity/Calm	Envy	Melancholy
5	Transparency	Non-attachment	Greed	Stinginess
6	Faith	Courage	Fear	Cowardice
7	Wisdom/Plan	Sobriety	Gluttony	Planning
8	Truth	Innocence	Lust	Vengeance

Enneagram of the Ego Ideals

9 Comfort/Harmony (Nines need to be peaceful and unobtrusive)
1 Perfection/Righteousness (Ones need to be good and perfect)
2 Helpfulness/Giving (Twos need to be helpful and self-sacrificing)
3 Success/Achievement (Threes need to be successful and efficient)
4 Originality/Specialness (Fours need to be original and refined)
5 Knowledge/Understanding (Fives need to be observant and wise)
6 Safety/Security (Sixes need to be on guard and loyal)
7 Imagination/Enjoyment (Sevens need to be joyful and enthusiastic)
8 Strength/Aggression (Eights need to be in control and assertive)

The ego ideal is the summation of all positive behaviours. It's a vision of optimal functioning – the belief that there is an ideal way to function and appear.

Enneagram of Avoidances

9 Conflict
1 Wrongness
2 Neediness
3 Failure
4 Despair
5 Emptiness
6 Deviance
7 Pain
8 Weakness

Each type has something they want to avoid in life. The compulsions of our type maintain self-image and enable avoidance. We avoid what challenges us to grow. For example, the avoidance of the perfectionist (type One) is anger. They avoid anger because you cannot be perfect and angry (in their fantasy). The avoided anger blocks the perfectionist on the journey to wholeness.

Vulnerabilities

Aside from the Virtues and Vices, Fixations and Holy Ideas, each type has a vulnerability (sore spot or fundamental fear) as well as a defence mechanism (the self-protective strategy we employ to shield ourselves against criticism, conflict, or pressure to change), which are activated when confronted by our blind spots. They are:

Type	Vulnerability	Defence Mechanism
9	Conflict	Narcotisation/introjection
1	Criticism	Reaction formation/projective identification
2	Being unloved	Repression
3	Being worthless	Identification
4	Looking ordinary	Sublimation
5	Being unprepared	Isolation/compartmentalisation
6	Being unprepared	Projection
7	Limitation	Reframing/rationalisation
8	Being vulnerable	Denial

Instincts and Fears

There are three groups of instincts, together with their three primordial fears:

Self-Preservative (SP)	'I'	Fear of not surviving
Sexual (SX)	'Us'	Fear of being unwanted
Social (SO)	'We'	Fear of not belonging

Instincts are biological drives in humans for self-preservation, social belonging, and one-on-one bonding. They profoundly influence our being in the world. The instincts blend with the nine types to create three distinct subtypes, where the core type and dominant instinctual drive come together to create an even more specific focus of attention and expression. We have all three survival instincts, but one will be dominant, another secondary, and the third one will be repressed. For example, in the animal kingdom, there will be:

1 Nesting (SP)
2 Mating (SX)
3 Herding (SO)

The three instincts can be described as:

• Preserving
• Merging
• Navigating

The Self-Preservative instinct revolves around safety and security concerns, avoiding danger, maintaining a sense of structure, and having sufficient resources to meet the demands of the environment and other people. The Sexual instinct focuses a person on impacting their environment through intense experiences and relationships. Energy and excitement drive them to others in terms of procuring deep interpersonal connections and meaningful experiences. The Social instinct focuses a person on status, social standards, hierarchy, and belonging in groups. The subtype is the overlay of the instinct onto the core type (the instinctual overlay creates the subtype). Thus, we can say that:

$$\text{Type} + \text{Instinct} = \text{Subtype (general)}$$

$$\text{Passion} + \text{Instinct} = \text{Subtype (more specific)}$$

There are twenty-seven (i.e., 9×3) subtypes, as we have seen. Within each set of three subtypes, one instinct will pull us in a different direction (the opposite behaviourally to our core type) creating countertypes. If, for example, the Passion (Vice) is gluttony (which it is for the Seven), then sacrifice will be the countertype. In types 1, 5, and 6, the Sexual instinct is the countertype; in types 2, 3, and 4, the instinct of Self-Preservation is the countertype; and in types 7, 8, and 9, the Social instinct is the countertype. The system is further layered in terms of the *wings*, that is, those types existing on either side of one's main type. Thus, a Seven will have wings 6 and 8.

Challenges

Each type has an emotional challenge linked to its three centres.

Types	Emotional Issues	Examples
Action: 1, 9, 8	Anger, control, autonomy	Ones internalise anger; Nines have a conflicted relationship with anger; Eights externalise anger.
Feeling: 4, 3, 2	Shame, self-esteem, acceptance	Fours internalise shame; Threes have a complicated relationship to shame; Twos externalise their shame.
Thinking: 5, 6, 7	Fear, anxiety, cynicism	Fives internalise their fear; Sixes are conflicted about their anxiety; Sevens externalise their fear (by focusing on the future).

The three options are:

- Internalised action: turns inward
- Externalised action: turns outward (acts out)
- Contradicted: confused/withdrawn

Stress Points

Stress is a slippery slope toward addiction. Each type can disintegrate under stress leading them to behave like another type in their most dysfunctional incarnation. Each number on the Enneagram has two lines attached to it: one for stress and one for security. The lines help us understand when we are stressed, how we act under stress, and show better ways of handling stress.

They are known as the lines of integration and disintegration, so that when a Seven, to take one example, is stretched/stressed they move to One and adopt the characteristics of a One (the strict perfectionist), and when secure/safe the Seven will go to Five (the quiet specialist). An average-to-unhealthy One under stress will behave (eventually) like an average-to-unhealthy Four; an average-to-unhealthy Four will act out their stress like an average-to-unhealthy Two. You remain your core type but may experience points when you adopt the characteristics of a type on the other side of your line.

- One goes to Four – The critical, judgemental, perfectionistic One becomes moody, melancholic, irritable, and withdrawn. But by using the healthier traits of a Four, they can become creative, aesthetic, and introspective. Ones need to get more in touch with nature and their feelings.
- Two goes to Eight – The prideful, manipulative, martyrish Two becomes aggressive, demanding, domineering, argumentative, controlling, and blunt. Or they can use some of the healthier aspects of the Eight and get more in touch with their own needs, becoming more decisive and protective. Twos need to give themselves the time for self-care and do some activities alone.
- Three goes to Nine – The vain, validatory, inauthentic, needy Three becomes complacent, apathetic, self-doubting, disengaged, and retreating. They can become instead open-hearted and non-judgemental. The Three needs to connect with people heart to heart.
- Four goes to Two – The moody, temperamental, withdrawn Four can become a people-pleaser, buying others' love and flattering them, or they can become friendly and loving. The Four needs to work with those in need, volunteering for some service.
- Five goes to Seven – The withdrawn, cynical, stingy Five becomes indulgent, distracted, dissatisfied, or gets more adventurous, imaginative, confident, and future-oriented. When stressed, Fives need to indulge moderately and do fun things.
- Six goes to Three – The self-doubting, anxious, highly vigilant Six becomes dishonest, busy, and image-conscious, or they create goals and get optimistically motivated. Stressed Sixes need to talk to trusted friends.
- Seven goes to One – The unfocused, indulgent, escapist Seven becomes rigid, perfectionistic, pessimistic, and angry, or they begin to look at their problems rationally without reframing and feel all emotions, not just pleasurable ones. Stressed Sevens need to explore their feelings and finish plans.
- Eight goes to Five – The controlling, rebellious, intimidating Eight becomes secretive, withdrawn, cynical, stingy, critical, and detached. The hope is that they will look at the problem objectively and observe their emotions. The Eight needs physical activity as a release for pent-up energy.
- Nine goes to Six – The indecisive, passive–aggressive forgetful Nine becomes anxious, suspicious, overcommitted, worried, and depressive, or he does what needs to be done and sticks to routine and commits to self-care. Nines need to honour other peoples' suggestions more.

These lines are fluid not fixed – dynamic and developmental – so that a Seven, for example, can move to both One and Five when stressed and introject aspects pertaining to both types.

The Enneagram shows a way out of the maze, of the labyrinth of our ego: from being trapped and held in a trance and having a frozen and fixated relationship to our type to a more aware, freer stance. Each type is connected to two others by lines of stress (stretch) and security (release). These lines represent alternative dimensions, opportunities for more balanced behaviour. Moving along the lines represents a significant shift in perspective, which enables one to step out of typical and entrenched reactive patterns. The IEQ9 Enneagram test shows a 'Strain Profile' which reflects and reveals how much pressure one is presently under; the results are subjective and time-sensitive. In the Enneagram symbol, the line pointing *towards* the core type represents the direction of stretch (challenge), guiding clients to access the higher and healthier aspects of their line. The line pointing *from* one's core type represents the direction of security (possibility). Moving along this line one explores the higher aspect of the connected type which opens the door to relieving stress and increasing resilience. So, these lines of integration and disintegration are not static; they are not ineluctable patterns of collapse to the low (unhealthy) side of one connected point or conversely to accessing through integration the higher side of a healthy connected point, which the terms themselves imply. To spell this out, a Seven when stressed, as we said, moves to One (becoming a strict perfectionist) and when integrated moves to Five (becoming a quiet specialist), *but* it's just as possible to integrate the higher side of the so-called disintegration point or take on the less useful qualities of their 'integration' point. The aim is to connect with the higher aspect of *each* connected type, not the fixated side. The release point tends to offer relief from strain just as the stretch point tends to take someone out of their comfort zone. It's the grit in the oyster that becomes a pearl. Sometimes stress brings out the best in us, and at other times, the worst. When stressed, it's as if a switch is flicked and we act like someone else.

Type	Release Point	Stretch Point
One	Seven	Four
Two	Four	Eight
Three	Six	Nine
Four	One	Two
Five	Eight	Seven
Six	Nine	Three
Seven	Five	One
Eight	Two	Five
Nine	Three	Six

- What stresses the One: being around lazy or non-dependable people; not living up to their own expectations; feeling they're carrying all the responsibility; being taken for granted; hypocrisy; apathy; unpunctuality; messiness.

- What stresses the Two: having too much time alone; feeling unloved; saying yes to too many things; not getting affirmation or appreciation; feeling left out; being around emotionally unattuned people; not feeling needed.
- What stresses the Three: not seeing progress in relation to goal setting; feeling like a failure or incompetent; not being acknowledged; losing; being compared to successful people; feeling worthless; not being challenged; being around people who lack vision and verve.
- What stresses the Four: having to go along with the crowd; too many external responsibilities; feeling misunderstood and criticised or micromanaged; being forced to follow rules and regulations; not being able to make creative decisions; having to put on a happy face when they don't feel like it; living in squalid surroundings; feeling stymied or blocked.
- What stresses the Five: not getting enough alone time; being barged in on; neglect; feeling displaced from the physical world; being overwhelmed by dark thoughts; not finding a niche for themselves; feeling that life is meaningless; isolation and lack of connection/communication.
- What stresses the Six: undependable people; disorder; chaos; not having support; catastrophising; feeling unsafe; lack of structure; burnout; wishy-washy behaviour; making mistakes.
- What stresses the Seven: being micromanaged; not having enough personal freedom; lack of free time; being cooped up; restrictions; excessive responsibilities; boredom and routine; nitty-gritty detail; financial problems; lack of loyalty in friendship.
- What stresses the Eight: feeling out of control; having to be a follower; infringements on their autonomy; failure; not seeing progress; vapid people; having to sugar-coat things and having to play it safe; corruption; not being challenged sufficiently.
- What stresses the Nine: conflict in their environment; being with people who are making a scene or a claim; being passed over; saying yes to things they don't want to do; dealing with peer pressure; losing relationships; suppressing anger; having too many demands placed on their time.

These tell-tale signs are worth watching for, as there can be a thin line between stress and addiction.

Recovery

The aim here is to leverage the similarities between the Twelve Step recovery and the Enneagram for an integral programme of psycho-spirituality. Transformation occurs at the psychological and spiritual level. What are you addicted to? Answer: more. The ego craves and clings and chases. It is addictive at its very core. The Enneagram works from the inside out (our motivations) rather than the outside in (our behaviours), as we said, and this makes it deeper than any other so-called personality system. Any change or growth will involve three steps:

- Awareness – appraisal of what's not working.
- Acceptance – realisation that the new behaviour and attitude will take time.
- Action – daily disciplined practice.

In the very first step of Alcoholics Anonymous (A.A.), we become aware we are powerless; we accept this, and we decide to proceed with a plan of action. We name the ego addiction. The Big Book says the aim is to help the attendees discover 'a chink in the walls their ego has built, through which the light of reason can shine' (*Alcoholics Anonymous*, p. 46). In the Enneagram, our compulsive behaviours are called the Passions (when our feeling centre is out of sync), and Fixations is the name given to when our thinking is out of alignment with our Holy Ideas. Our essence gets covered up with a dominant coping strategy around the body (instinctual), head (thinking), and heart (feeling) centres. The circle encompassing the Enneagram types/numbers represents unity/ oneness/wholeness, as it does in the recovery symbol. Bill W was reportedly a Three on the Enneagram. We can see the personality types as various addictions. The Enneagram shows our ego traps and a roadmap for change, as we transition from our Passions (defects/shortcomings) to our Virtues (essential, non-addictive qualities).

A.A. Principles

Earlier, we listed the Enneagram of Virtues. The equivalent twelve principles in A.A. are:

 1 Honesty
 2 Hope
 3 Faith
 4 Courage
 5 Integrity
 6 Willingness
 7 Humility
 8 Compassion
 9 Balance (Justice)
10 Perseverance
11 Spirituality
12 Service

We have traits from all nine types, but one will be dominant. Our personality type is stable. Our passions are our ego addictions. They make us lose sight of our Virtues – these bring us back to our essence, return us to our centre.

We repeat our old patterns in our Passions. Hopefully, we can practice our unique Virtues too. If the former suggests our addictions, the latter signals ways we can become free. Freedom is ultimately overcoming our personality fixations and compulsions. Many of these will be the unaddressed and unacknowledged issues left over from childhood. Our Instincts arise from our body centre (reptilian or hindbrain), our Passions arise from our feeling centre (limbic system), and our Fixations arise from our thinking centre (the prefrontal cortex in the forebrain).

Instincts	Body/Gut	Reptilian brain
Passions	Feeling	Limbic system
Fixations	Thinking	Forebrain

So, we have three centres of intelligence:

Heart	Emotional intelligence (Twos, Threes, Fours)	EQ
Head	Cognitive intelligence (Fives, Sixes, Sevens)	IQ
Gut	Instinctual intelligence (Eights, Nines, Ones)	GQ

In a fight-or-flight or freeze situation, our instincts are activated first and faster than our feelings or thoughts. In the fourth step of A.A., we take an inventory of what the Enneagram calls our social, security, and sexual instincts:

- Resentments (social instinct)
- Fears (security or self-preservative instinct)
- Sex conduct (our sexual instinct)

The instincts are powerful body-based forces; they represent the primal strategy of how best to survive.

Instinct	Associated Energy
Self-preservative	Withdrawing, avoiding, protecting
Sexual	Approaching, acquiring, fending off
Social	Connecting, including, relating

The way to bring the energies into balance so we can live harmoniously with ourselves, and others, is to redistribute their energy. Here, we take a portion of our investment away from our dominant instinct and give it to our repressed instinct.

The Big Book mentions that 'the main problems of the alcoholic [addicted person] centres in his mind, rather than in his body' (*Alcoholics Anonymous*,

p. 23). These obsessions of the mind are mental fixations, according to the Enneagram. When we lose touch with our essence, we develop lower mental patterns called fixations which are filters that limit seeing things from another angle. We can put it this way:

• Body or gut-based – Instincts
• Feeling or heart-based – Passions
• Thinking or mind (head)-based – Fixations

The instincts show the first differentiation from essence, the passions are the second layer, and the fixations are the final egoic coping strategy. Feelings and thoughts are not isolated from each other; rather, they influence each other. By contrast with our Passions and Fixations, our Holy Ideas connect us with the Higher Power (universal consciousness), which is the aim of A.A. recovery, Advaita, meditation, and the Enneagram.

Exercise: Thought patterns can cause disturbances and upset, so a useful technique is to pause and spot the 'hot thought'. We need to work on moving away from negative emotions and toxic thoughts. Let's look at four basic/primary emotions:

1 Happy
2 Sad
3 Fearful
4 Angry

Other emotions such as surprise can be seen as Happy + Fear (pleasant surprise) or Angry + Fear (if an unpleasant surprise). Feelings are an ever-changeable source of information. They are not objective facts in that they subjectively colour impressions and experiences we've had. Under anger may be fear; joy can cover fear; sadness can cover joy.

Steps 8 and 9 of A.A. require people to make amends to those whom they have hurt. Confronting our shadow sides and engaging with others constructively and compassionately is difficult.

There are four components of nonviolent communication which one can practice (see Jenner K in *The Enneagram for Recovery*, p. 113–114), in this regard:

1 Observations – no interpretive words, just the facts/descriptions.
2 Feelings – how we feel about what we observe.
3 Needs – the desires that are and are not being met.
4 Requests – for what we do want, not a demand.

We have all nine types in us. If we want to truly know ourselves, which is the foundation of all this work, we need to pay close attention to ourselves and to the architecture of the Enneagram. Each type has a wing (a neighbouring type) on each side so, for example, a 7 has a 6 and 8 wing (thus 7w6 and 7w8). At least one of your wings will be within your same centre of body, heart, or head intelligence.

Wings

The eighteen wing types are (see Jenner K, *The Enneagram for Recovery*, p. 124–128):

- Type 9w8: The Comfort Seeker
- Type 9w1: The Dreamer
- Type 1w9: The Idealist
- Type 1w2: The Advocate
- Type 2w1: The Servant
- Type 2w3: The Host
- Type 3w2: The Star
- Type 3w4: The Professional
- Type 4w3: The Aristocrat
- Type 4w5: The Bohemian
- Type 5w4: The Iconoclast
- Type 5w6: The Problem Solver
- Type 6w5: The Defender
- Type 6w7: The Buddy
- Type 7w6: The Entertainer
- Type 7w8: The Realist
- Type 8w7: Maverick
- Type 8w9: The Bear

These neighbouring wings influence but do not change the core type. A person doesn't take on the motivations of the wings, but by leaning into them he can widen his perspective and increase his emotional and behavioural repertoire. Ideally, we will access both wings, each of which will offer its own resources. (We shift from one wing to another depending on circumstance and context.) We need balanced access to both.

- 9 accessing an 8 wing can become more assertive and take charge; accessing a 1 wing, can get to know boundaries more.
- 1 accessing a 9 wing can embrace multiple viewpoints; accessing a 2 wing can focus more on people.
- 2 accessing a 1 wing can become more discerning; accessing a 3 wing can become more of a leader.
- 3 accessing a 2 wing can motivate others; accessing a 4 wing can begin to show and share feelings.

- 4 accessing a 3 wing can focus more on work; accessing a 5 wing can set clear boundaries.
- 5 accessing a 4 wing can connect to deeper feelings; accessing a 6 wing can connect and commit.
- 6 accessing a 5 wing can practice self-containment; accessing a 7 wing can have spontaneous fun.
- 7 accessing a 6 wing can face their fears; accessing an 8 wing can ground their action.
- 8 accessing a 7 wing can lighten up; accessing their 9 wing can combine strength with kindness.

It is now thought that the wings are the flavouring, but the subtypes are more important than the wings. Instinct creates the subtype, not the wings. Furthermore, we may distinguish three social styles (how I get what I want). These are called Hornevian social styles (of interaction) as they are influenced by psychoanalyst Karen Horney's thinking. Each type has a tendency to:

- Move toward (give in)
- Move against (fight)
- Move away (keep to oneself)

- The Assertives are types 3, 7, 8 (move against).
- The Compliants are types 1, 2, 6 (move toward).
- The Withdrawns are types 4, 5, 9 (move away).

If Assertives are aggressive and expansive, Withdrawns are detached and resigned, while Compliants are abiding and idealistic. The compliant is the self-effacing solution, the aggressive is the self-expansive solution, and the detached is the resignation solution. The Hornevians are social styles – they're about how to get what you want (and are not linked to the centres). For example, if we take the Withdrawn types, which are Fours, Fives, and Nines, there will be a:

- Feeling Withdrawn (Enneatype 4)
- Thinking Withdrawn (Enneatype 5)
- Acting Withdrawn (Enneatype 9)

The objective, as always, is to seek balance and also to work on the integration of heart, head, and hands (body) as, during the course of the Twelve Steps, we return to our essence by awareness, and we move from Passions and Fixations to Virtues and Holy Ideas, through painful growth. The author of *The Enneagram for Recovery* provides an amusing summary of each type's unique slogan at the conclusion of the book (see Jenner K, *The Enneagram for Recovery*, p. 150):

Type	Bumper Sticker
1	Live and let live
2	Humility is not thinking less of yourself, but thinking of yourself less
3	To thine own Self be true
4	Attitude of gratitude
5	Oh, lighten up!
6	Face everything and recover
7	One day at a time
8	Easy does it!
9	First things first

The Great Exit

Redemption involves less ego and more essence. Each type has his/her own work to do on moving from addiction/compulsion/fixation to fullness of life.

- Ones – If they accept the world as it is instead of standing against it and seeking to correct it, they will be at peace and achieve that serenity for which they long. Ones are invited to see that everyone is already perfect in their essence and that the present moment is perfect too.
- Twos – If they accept the fact that they are not as indispensable to others as they believe, their pride will give way to humility. Twos are invited to stop trying to control the universe and rescue others and acknowledge instead that other forces are at play.
- Threes – If they connect with hope, they begin to believe that the world is generous, and they experience the joy of who they are rather than relying on their image. The universe operates according to its own laws, and this natural rhythm will continue without the Three's assistance. Threes will realise that they are part of something bigger that works through the creation.
- Fours – If they begin to see the positive as well as the negative in equal measure, they will achieve equanimity. When they cease comparing themselves with others their envy will fade away. They are invited to know that they are connected to the Source and are not isolated or separate but part of a creative flow. They are special regardless.
- Fives – If they just begin to realise that they will understand the world better by participating in it, they will become less detached and know their resources will always be replenished if they would just trust and take only what they need. They are invited to become aware that there is a more universal power of knowing (omniscience) and true wisdom comes from engagement with all of life's vicissitudes.

- Sixes – If they only knew that their safety and security fears were largely self-created, they would know courage and peace. No longer held captive by them, they would question their own assumptions and act without deference to authority. They are invited to know the universe takes care of them anyway. Having faith involves this primordial trust in the goodness of essential nature.
- Sevens – If they could relinquish their gluttonous hunger and temper their insatiable need for stimulation, they would find sober joy, anchoring themselves in the present. They are invited to slow down and see that all things work to a (divine) providential plan in the ongoing unfoldment of reality.
- Eights – If they could move into innocence, they would become more open-hearted and experience the nuances of life without jaded expectations. They are invited to step beyond their desires and interpretations to see universal truth.
- Nines – If they would move out of inertia and discover their own intention they would begin to live more fully and completely. They are invited to see that even when they lose sight of themselves, they are loved just for who they are.

All types, with Enneagram practice as well as meditation, can reach the state of alignment, of being in sync with the Self, rather than the ego impostor. In terms of the three centres of intelligence, this will result in being:

- Grounded in the body (alive).
- Connected to the heart (open).
- Attaining a quiet (still and spacious) mind.

We travel the path from no awareness to fixation, from adaptive self-awareness to true transformative self-awareness to liberation (enlightenment). When we get triggered, my emotional passions are activated, and the defence mechanisms come into play. But when we become aware, we can choose a different pattern of behaviour. The aim is to wake up from trance; spot our biases; become aware of our fears, vices, and defences; balance our centres; understand our motivations; work with our core type and subtypes; and find release, security, and harmony.

Idealised Self-Images

Each type has an idealised self-image and a blind spot.

Type	Idealised Self-Image	Blind Spot
Ones	I am good, right, perfect	Feeling like a bad person
Twos	I am helpful, generous, giving	Feeling worthless/not needed
Threes	I am competent, efficient, successful	Failing/being incapable

Fours	I am original, authentic, different	Being ordinary
Fives	I am knowledgeable, perceptive, thoughtful	Not having enough/being foolish
Sixes	I am loyal, faithful, obedient	Being unprepared for threats
Sevens	I am energetic, enthusiastic, OK	Restrictions/limitations
Eights	I am powerful, effective, adaptable	Feeling vulnerable/weak
Nines	I am agreeable, affable, and peaceful	Being in conflict

The hope is that we see our Vices – those fixated, limiting, distorted world-views – upfront and move towards the balancing forces of our Virtues – to more positive, healthier possibilities. It is a journey of integration, of individuation.

Type	Vice	Virtue
Ones	Anger	Serenity
Twos	Pride	Humility
Threes	Deceit	Hope
Fours	Envy	Equanimity
Fives	Avarice	Detachment
Sixes	Doubt	Faith
Sevens	Gluttony	Sobriety
Eights	Lust	Innocence
Nines	Self-forgetfulness	Right action

Going forward, it is hoped that every Twelve Step recovery programme will include/incorporate these three highly compatible, core ingredients:

• Contemplative practice (Ignatian, Christian Mediation, Transcendental Meditation, or Centering Prayer, for example)
• Enneagram work (as a central feature/aspect for all addicted subjects)
• Journalling

A truly integral model would include weekly A.A. meetings (the Twelve Step programme of recovery), daily contemplative practice, journalling, and ongoing Enneagram coaching. And Enneagram coaching, for its part, would encourage the practice of meditation as a key adjunct to its approach. 'The Enneagram's practical spirituality aligns so well with what we're trying to accomplish in recovery' (Jenner K, *The Enneagram for Recovery*, p. 150), as the addicted person travels on his journey from slavery to sobriety.

Russ Hudson, the eminent Enneagram expert, said, 'Inner work is what the Enneagram is for' (webinar, Enneagram Global Summit, December 12, 2021). He argued that there are three aspects to such work:

- Cultivation of Presence (soul-making; to increase our capacity to be present and available to Presence in the body, mind, and heart)
- Working through (one's psychological patterns, wounds, traumas – healing is part of the spiritual path)
- Practice (daily life as the laboratory and monastery)

Chapter 10

An Ignatian Interlude

St Ignatius of Loyola

Before his cannonball moment and subsequent conversion, he had what could only be described as high piety and low morals. There were rumours he had a bastard child; he was punctilious about his appearance, anxious to please the opposite sex, daring in gallantry, fearing nothing. Vanity and vainglory were his vices. One Jesuit lists his characterological traits thus: gambling addictions, sexual promiscuity, conceit, touchiness, quick temper (see William Watson, SJ, *Sacred Story*, p. 12). He suffered early maternal deprivation, which was a probable contributing factor to his phallic narcissism and addictions. He identified his later religious scruples as rooted in pride – his core sin. Christian tradition has variously described pride, vainglory, or narcissism as the chief vice. So Ignatius, through an examen of his consciousness, pinpoints the root cause of his addictions. He looks to God for graces, admitting to himself that he can't save himself. Thus there is the initial confrontation with his root 'sin' (seen by him in these religious terms, which the Enneagram calls a Passion), the effort to control it by sheer force of will, despair (sometimes suicidal) at not being able to, coupled with his desire to change and embark on a spiritual journey, admitting his powerlessness (aka Alcoholic Anonymous [A.A.]), surrendering prideful actions, and allowing the divine to shape his story. He also experienced a trio of near-death experiences (in 1522, 1532, and 1550). His life seems to follow the threefold mystical path of purgation, illumination, and union.

St Ignatius's book *The Spiritual Exercises* had as its purpose the conquest of self (ego) and the ordering (regulation) of one's life. He named his addictions as false lovers offering only a chimera of happiness. The white and black noise that worked on him throughout his life pushed and pulled his thoughts, feelings, and deeds in two different directions – one life-giving (which he called 'consolations'), the other life-destroying (which he called 'desolations'). He

DOI: 10.4324/9781003422570-11

saw addictions as anaesthesia, as counterfeit peace-providers. The advice he gave in *The Spiritual Exercises* was that upon immediately rising in the morning we should resolve to guard against a particular sin/defect/fault/addiction, and if one falls into the addictive behaviour, then ask for the grace to make amends and avoid it in the future. He suggests sifting through the day in the examen, recalling one's thoughts, feelings, and actions from the day. The objective is to spot the miscreant, to trace and track the thought-feeling that gave rise to the temptation.

Ignatian Checklist

An Ignatian checklist suggests itself for the purpose of daily discernment:

- Identification of the root vice.
- Awareness upon rising of the named addiction.
- Pauses during the day to take note of it and how it is developing, deepening, or diminishing.
- Marking in a journal what one seeks to reform and charting the progress made over days and weeks.
- Conscious attention to one's thoughts, words, and deeds during the course of a day.
- Seeing the source of one's stress in life events and traumas that can act as accomplices, spotting one's egoic personality patterns and passions at play.

The aim is integrated spiritual–psychological healing. It's an 'emotional *archaeology*', in Watson's words (Watson, *Sacred Story*, p. 65). Ignatius wished to be contemplative in action, living in the *sacrament of the present moment* (named as such by Jean-Pierre de Caussade, SJ). Ignatius anchored his consciousness in the present, tracing the contours of consolation and desolation, enjoying also 'consolation without previous cause', as he called it (which is grace). Greed, materialism, anger, sexual lust, gambling, and violent temper were all things Ignatius had to battle with and overcome. He saw them for what they were: enemies of true human nature. Addiction is often a misguided attempt to relieve stress. Greed, gluttony, and pride are deep-rooted in our hearts, souls, and biochemical/psychological make-up. Gabor Maté proposes a five-level strategy which reflects a strong spiritual acumen, which aligns well with St Ignatius (see Watson, *Sacred Story*, p. 91):

- Relabel
- Reattribute
- Refocus
- Revalue
- Recreate

The method/template described by Watson, rejigging Maté, is:

- *Declare* to Christ/the Absolute/Oneself the specific addiction or destructive compulsion as a false lover.
- *Describe* to Christ/the Absolute/Oneself the specific addiction or destructive compulsion as coming from the enemy of your human nature.
- *Descend* with Christ/the Absolute/Oneself into your memory to 'see' and 'feel' your first experience of this specific addiction or compulsion, asking Him to compassionately reveal the stress fractures, loneliness, and wounds in your heart it promised to satisfy.
- *Denounce*, with Christ/the Absolute/Oneself, as you witness the addiction or destructive compulsion for its ruinous effect in your life.
- *Decide* for Christ/the Absolute/Oneself to heal this wound; diffuse the stress, anxiety, and fear feeding it; and transform its damaging effects on your life, paying particular attention to the trinity of emotions – anger, fear (anxiety-stress), and grief (see Watson, *Sacred Story*, p. 92).

Journalling

Recovery requires disconnecting from false lovers and reconnecting with what is eternal and everlasting. Watson recommends identifying ten neuralgic events and persons from your past and 'watching' these events/persons dispassionately, 'feeling' them until they reveal in your heart the reason(s) why they create pain, stress, and discomfort. Here we invite conscious awareness of significant memories that are a symbol and sign of blockages preventing emotional and spiritual growth. 'Graced awareness is sought to remember, name, and perceive any destructive spiritual and psychological events whose injury to one's human nature reverberates to the present day' (Watson, *Sacred Story*, p. 107). This particular substance may provide momentary pleasure, but I pay attention to the *afterglow*, to how I am feeling in its wake. I focus on why I was anxious and why I was inspired. We need to listen to our addictions and write about them in a notebook: they are obstacles to living in freedom and with (ordered) desire. Watson recommends listing when you think you are *o*ccasionally, *fre*quently, or *c*onstantly ensnared by the 'enemy' (as Ignatius calls it) of our human nature (colloquially, we hear the expression: 'you're your own worst enemy') (see Watson, *Sacred Story*, p. 173). Thus, for example, I can take note of how mildly, moderately, or seriously the addictions in question ensnare me:

- TV – Occasionally
- Drinking – Frequently
- Pornography – Constantly

A spiritual diagnostic will also take into account the persons/events that not only initiated fear, anger, or grief but also gratitude, hope, or love.

Exercise: List ten persons/issues/events that initiated fear, anger, or grief, and then ten that initiated gratitude, hope, or love (see Watson, *Sacred Story*, pp. 180–181).

Person/Issue/Event	Fear, Anger, or Grief
1	1
2	2
3	3
4	4
5	5
6	6
7	7
8	8
9	9
10	10

Person/Issue/Event	Gratitude, Hope, or Love
1	1
2	2
3	3
4	4
5	5
6	6
7	7
8	8
9	9
10	10

One must learn to see one's life in terms of a *narrative* unity, as the philosophers Alasdair MacIntyre and Paul Ricoeur call it – it is the conception of life as a quest in search of meaning.

Chapter 11

Platonic Ethics, St. Benedict, and the Law of *Dharma*

Plato's Virtues

The point was made earlier in the book that temperance is the virtue most needed in addiction. And it is the point of the Enneagram, as we saw, to show us our virtues and the path leading from vice to virtue.

Western philosophical ethics began with the great Greek triumvirate of Socrates, Plato, and Aristotle. Plato propounded the famous four cardinal virtues in *The Republic*:

- Wisdom
- Courage (fortitude)
- Temperance (moderation)
- Justice

Plato adds holiness in the *Protagoras*. 'Cardinal' comes from *cardo* meaning 'hinge' (i.e., central). Plato will stress the unity of the virtues. They all interrelate. This is important lest one propose a syllogism thus: Courage is a virtue, the Nazis are courageous, therefore, the Nazis are virtuous. Courage can't be abstracted from wisdom, justice, and temperance. Virtues cannot exist independently, and the opposite of a virtue is a vice. To the four cardinal virtues, Christianity added three theological virtues: faith, hope, and love. If the moral virtues are acquired, the supernatural virtues are infused in the soul through grace. For Plato, the philosopher-king will create a just society/state: the movement will be from *psyche* to *polis*.

Franklin's Moral Checklist

Benjamin Franklin, the polymath founding father of the United States, provided his own moral checklist, which featured temperance in the number one place:

- Temperance – eat not to dullness, drink not to elevation.
- Silence – speak not but what benefits others; avoid trifling conversation.

DOI: 10.4324/9781003422570-12

- Order – let everything have its place; let each part of your business have its time.
- Resolution – perform without fail what you resolve.
- Frugality – make no expense but to do good to others; waste nothing.
- Industry – lose no time; be employed in usefulness; cut off all unnecessary action.
- Sincerity – use no deceit; speak accordingly.
- Justice – wrong none, by doing injury or by omission of benefits.
- Moderation – avoid extremes.
- Cleanliness – tolerate no uncleanness in body, clothes, or habitation.
- Tranquillity – be not disturbed by trifles.
- Chastity – rarely use venery but for health or offspring.
- Humility – imitate Jesus and Socrates.

Such virtues appear similar across time and countries – a cross-cultural convergence is at play as we are talking of universal principles. In *A Short Treatise on the Great Virtues*, French philosopher André Comte-Sponville enumerates his list, which also includes temperance:

Politeness	Simplicity
Fidelity	Tolerance
Prudence	Purity
Temperance	Gentleness
Courage	Good faith
Justice	Humour
Generosity	Love
Compassion	Mercy
Gratitude	Humility

Humility is an interesting virtue as one won't find it in Roman and Greek philosophy; this virtue would have to wait until the advent of Christianity. The good man is humble. He is humble because he sees himself as nothing and therefore can see other things as they are. Roman virtues included abundance (prosperity for all), humour, courtesy, clemency (mercy), tenacity, frugality, humanity (refinement), joy (gladness), justice, prudence, truthfulness (*veritas* – the mother of virtues), and trust (the root of all virtue). The key equation is this: *arete* (virtue) leads to *eudaimonia* (sustainable, spiritual happiness/ flourishing).

The Four Foundations

The good person is the happy person. We may distinguish four fundamentals (dimensions of human experience) – for sustaining ethical excellence in all we do:

1 The intellectual dimension – truth
2 The aesthetic dimension – beauty
3 The moral dimension – goodness
4 The spiritual dimension – unity

Thus: the transcendentals of the True, the Good, the Beautiful (metaphysical not physical), and the One.

Meanwhile, Christianity adopted Plato's list and it also gave us the Ten Commandments. The Decalogue outlines various prescriptions: Thou shalt not kill, steal, commit adultery, etc. The Golden Rule: Do unto others what you would have them do unto you. A slightly different version is Confucius's: 'What you do not want done to yourself, do not do to others'. If wisdom is a form of understanding about how we ought to live, virtue is the habit of acting in accordance with such wisdom.

Aristotelian Ethics

For Aristotle, virtue is the midpoint between an excess (too much) and a deficiency (too little). To give an example of the Golden Mean in relation to the virtue of courage:

Excess	Virtue	Deficiency
Rashness	Courage	Cowardice

Human excellence is the art of character. Character is the art of practising the four cardinal virtues. Aristotle also argued for four intellectual virtues:

1 *Episteme* (knowledge)
2 *Phronesis* (practical wisdom)
3 *Techne* (technical skill/know-how)
4 *Sophia* (philosophical wisdom)

Let's explore each of the four cardinal virtues in the hierarchical order which Plato gave them.

Practical Wisdom

Prudence or practical wisdom is the ability to discern the appropriate course of action to be taken in a given situation. Prudence is right reason, the ability to judge correctly what is right and wrong, practical intelligence/life experience, open-mindedness, curiosity, lifelong learning, perspective. Prudence is the mould and mother of the other cardinal virtues (assigned by Plato to the rulers). Prudence is knowledge of reality and realisation of the good. It is the measure of justice, fortitude, and temperance. It informs the other virtues. Prudence is about making the right decisions, not being judgemental; it's discretion, good judgement, understanding priorities, and anticipation. A prudent person responds; he doesn't react. He is not driven by hasty decisions. The symbols of prudence are a book, a scroll, and a mirror.

Temperance

Temperance is restraint of our desires, right measure, self-control/discipline, moderation. It is common to all but associated with the producing class in Plato's republic such as farmers and craftsmen. The opposite of temperance is tempest, temper. Moderation is freedom. Temperance can be summed up as 'nothing to excess'; it's the balance of being (e.g., work–life), self-control (e.g., sticking to a diet, limiting your media consumption). Temperance consists in realising we're prone to pursuing pleasure and addictions. Its symbol is the wheel, the bridle and the reins, and the water and wine in two jugs.

Plato's *Charmides* is a dialogue on the topic of temperance. Charmides was Plato's uncle on his mother's side. Socrates's other interlocutor was Critias, a first cousin of Charmides and Plato's mother. Critias was also one of the Thirty Tyrants. Temperance in this dialogue involves a sense of dignity, decorum, and self-command. Charmides is said to be a beautiful boy, thoughtful, modest, and self-possessed. He is depicted as being beautiful both in body and in character, a wrestler who is famed too for his temperance. For Socrates, the soul is the source of (bodily) health, and one cures the soul through various 'charms', which consist of beautiful words. It is the result of such words, we are told, that temperance arises in the soul (see Plato, *Charmides*, 157e). Temperance or restraint is the remedy for excess. According to Charmides, temperance involves doing everything in a quiet way; he views temperance as a sort of quietness. The quiet are temperate. And temperance is one of the most admirable things. Socrates disagrees with the former assessment while agreeing with the latter one. Charmides goes on to say that he thinks temperance must be a sort of modesty, one that produces shame in people. He now defines it as the doing of good things (see Plato, *Charmides*, 164e). Socrates interposes and maintains that temperance is knowing oneself and cites the Delphic inscriptions/injunctions: 'know thyself' and 'nothing too much'. By means of temperance, every household would be well-run and every city well-governed.

The same would be the case if temperance reigned in a man's soul. Temperance is, thus, 'a great good' and if you are possessed of this moral virtue, 'you are blessed' (Plato, *Charmides*, 176e). It is the virtue that is most needed in the addicted subject's soul, as he struggles to order his life to the Good.

Courage

Courage or fortitude is forbearance, strength of spirit, mettle, endurance, resilience, the ability to face fears, perseverance, steadiness in the face of obstacles. It is assigned by Plato to the warrior class and defined by him in *Laches* as 'wise endurance of the soul'. Courage is grace under pressure; it's about keeping going when things get tough (grace under grit), drive. And this too is needed by the addicted person. Its symbols are armour, a club, a tower, and a yoke.

Justice

For Plato, justice is outside the class system; it rules the proper relationships between the other three cardinal virtues. Prudence and justice are the virtues through which we decide what needs to be done; fortitude is the strength required to do it. Justice is the determination to give everyone their due; it is fairness, rights, loyalty, leadership. Justice is blind (not prejudiced by personal preferences) – consisting of fair treatment without bias or prejudice. Justice is right proportion, harmony. Its symbol is the sword, balance, the scales, and the crown.

Taken together (*integritas*/integral), the four cardinal virtues form the basis of moral goodness in the person. In the good life, we must watch out for the ego. Deploying the virtues boosts happiness. One's character strengths lead to subjective wellbeing and a sense of personal fulfilment (in the language of modern psychology). Martin Luther King Jr is a good example of a world-class leader who sought justice through love.

Plato leaves us with an interesting thought experiment: If you had the ring of the shepherd boy Gyges that made you invisible, what would you do? How would you act? If we could avoid detection and so had no fear of punishment, what would be some of the things you might want to carry out? The good man is not even tempted to act unjustly.

We can put the person in question through four moral tests:

- The *publicity* test: How would I feel if my contemplated activities were reported in the paper or on TV?
- The *mentor* test: How would I feel if my actions were seen by my most revered mentor?
- The *role model* test: What would the wise (my greatest role model) do here?
- The *mirror* test: If I do this, can I look at myself in the mirror and feel pride?

To have a full life, addiction-free, we need all four virtues working harmoniously in the soul. Arguably, though, none is more important for the addicted subject than temperance (followed by courage). Temperance is moderation and measure; it is self-restraint and helps us avoid extravagant excess. It is calmness and self-control.

Temperance derives from the Latin *tempero* meaning 'restraint'. It originally referred to the balancing and mixing of temperature. For Aristotle, temperance is the mean with regard to (bodily) pleasures, while for the Stoics it is the rational faculty. Socrates practised all the virtues; he both abstained and enjoyed. Later philosophers would follow a similar path in their philosophical reflections on the subject: Michel de Montaigne viewed temperance as self-governance which involved curbing rather than suppressing one's desires. In *Paradise Lost*, John Milton called it 'the rule of not too much'. Temperance enables us to quench 'the flabby licentiousness of a lecherous desire for pleasure' in Josef Pieper's felicitous phrase (Pieper, *A Brief Reader on the Virtues of the Human Heart*, p. 35). In positive psychology, temperance is defined to include four main character strengths:

- Forgiveness
- Humility
- Prudence
- Self-regulation

It is a virtue that is included in Buddhism, Hinduism, and Western and Eastern philosophy. The *Brihadaranyaka Upanishad* (verse 5.2.3) outlines three characteristics of a good and well-developed person:

- Self-restraint (*damah*)
- Compassion and love for all sentient life (*daya*)
- Charity (*daana*)

Finally, in relation to temperance, Marsilio Ficino (1433–1499), the Italian Renaissance neo-Platonist philosopher, provides a short commentary on Plato's dialogue, the *Charmides*, believing that Plato's language resembles 'a divine pronouncement ... flowing with the sweetness of nectar' (Ficino, *Gardens of Philosophy*, p. 4). Plato is priest, prophet, philosopher, and 'the Prince of eloquence' (Ficino, *Gardens of Philosophy*, p. 7). The Good, in this Platonic picture, consists in the practice of the virtues: wisdom, courage, justice, and temperance. Ficino begins by telling us that Socrates's purpose in the work is to encourage everyone to practice temperance, especially three groups of people:

- The young (because the medicine needs to be administered quickly before they develop diseases of the soul, such as intemperance).
- The noble (because true nobility is found in virtue).
- The beautiful (because they are more depraved than most and stand in need of medicine for their profligacy).

Temperance begins with the beauty of the body; from there, it moves to the health of the body, then to the beauty of the soul, 'which is the temperance of emotion, the moderation of movements' (Ficino, *Gardens of Philosophy*, p. 84). Temperance in the mind consists of a harmonious correspondence between the faculty of intelligence and all that is perceived. Justice (in the state, or the soul) is also a kind of temperance as it is an 'appropriate moderation' (Ficino, *Gardens of Philosophy*, p. 84). Ficino quotes a maxim of Pythagoras: measure is the best thing of all. Temperance (*sophrosyne*) is the preserver of prudence, one which drives the darkness of disturbances away, so that the mind becomes calmer. Wisdom and prudence accompany temperance – indeed, Plato often intends them to be included in the word 'temperance'. Temperance is harmonious modulation but difficult both to define and acquire, especially seeing as we have been nurtured in intemperance from our infancy. Temperance 'resides in deep stillness', Ficino contends, and is 'the hardest thing of all to find within the soul' (Ficino, *Gardens of Philosophy*, p. 88).

I mentioned humility earlier. St Benedict has what amounts to a twelve-step programme on the topic in chapter 7 of his *Rule*, titled 'Concerning Humility'. The addicted person will need a modest view of themselves, lest in arrogance they think they have finally conquered their addictions for good.

St Benedict on Humility

The Christian tradition has always taught that he who exalts himself will be humbled and the humbled shall be exalted. Humility is crucial in recovery, and we saw that it featured in the seventh step of Alcoholics Anonymous (A.A.).

Humility allows one to ask for help and to admit that one has a problem in the first place. Humility involves seeing oneself realistically, both one's strengths and limitations. Humility contrasts with hubris. *Humilitas* keeps us grounded, earthed, rooted, centred (*humus* = earth). Aidos, in Greek mythology, was the goddess of humility – that quality that restrained humans from wrongdoing. Humility gets annexed to temperance in the Catholic philosophical tradition. It is the virtue that consists in keeping oneself within one's bounds, according to Aquinas. For Immanuel Kant, humility is a meta-attitude that constitutes the moral agent's proper perspective on himself. In short, humility leads to heaven. If we imagine Jacob's ladder, which depicts angels going up and coming down, we can say that descending takes place by exaltation and ascending by humility (a certain kind of humiliation).

St Benedict (480–547) lived in sixth-century Italy when the Roman Empire was disintegrating – Rome had fallen to the barbarians in 410 and was sacked again in 455. As a young nobleman, Benedict left Nursia in Umbria to attend school in Rome but disgusted by life there he sought out solitude in a cave at Subiaco. Monks joined him over time and reluctantly he became Abbot, founding a monastery on the mountains above Cassino. Benedict called his *Rule* written for the monks 'a little rule for beginners'; it contained directions

for all aspects of the monastic life. These are Benedict's twelve steps to humility
– there is wisdom in his list for those living outside monastery walls:

- Keep the fear of God before your eyes, that is to say, awe, honour, reverence. Here we avoid self-will and disordered desires; we live under the divine watchfulness. God knows/searches our hearts and minds.
- The spiritual journey takes us from the ego as default and dysfunctional mode network (love of self, my will be done) to love of God (Thy will be done). Life is not just about the pleasure of fulfilling my base desires.
- Be obedient, that is to say, listen, especially to one's spiritual superiors.
- In obstacles, show patience; be faithful. Endure suffering (demonstrate resilience).
- Reveal in prayer any thoughts in the heart or deeds done; hope in God (confess and seek forgiveness).
- Be content with the lowest and most menial treatment, judging oneself as a 'worthless workman'. Realise you are unworthy and exist only because of God's great love.
- Believe in your unworthiness, in your inferiority.
- Carry out the common good (rather than seek to satiate individual interests); set the example.
- Restrain your tongue; talk less. Keep silence.
- Don't be so quickly moved to laughter (guffawing hysterically). Stop being so frivolous.
- Speak a few reasonable words (no idle chit-chat) calmly (*gravitas*) and don't be so noisy.
- Be humble in heart, always – in the monastery, garden, on the road, sitting or standing. Account for yourself, especially your sins (faults/vices).

Then and only then will humility become a habit – a cleansing agent of the soul, and one's second nature.

Ethics in Eastern Philosophy

The Vedas, for their part, list ten virtues. By way of conclusion, I would like to offer a brief ten-step Advaitin addition to the Twelve Steps as a blueprint for non-addicted living, followed by ten universal principles.

Dharma, which we came across earlier, is natural law, our purpose for being. The *Sanatana Dharma*, meaning 'eternal dharma' (order), is taken from the *Manu-smriti* (Laws of Manu), which is a book of the Hindu code and attributed to the legendary first man and lawgiver, Manu ('man' being human and *man* as in 'to think'/mind). In realising *dharma*, we realise freedom and our wellbeing. *Dharma* is our upliftment and salvation – a guide to living. Because *dharma* is temperance, it is the ultimate answer to addiction. Indeed, the 'temperance movement', begun in 1829, was dedicated to promoting moderation (and more often, complete abstinence) in the use of intoxicating liquor. There are ten aspects/applied principles of *dharma*, of truth and justice, each one of which brings us to enlightenment (Self-realisation):

1 Patience/Confidence/Courage (*Dhrh*)
2 Forgiveness/Tolerance (*Kshama*)
3 Temperance/Self-Control (*Dhama*)
4 Non-Stealing (*Asteya*)
5 Purity (*Shaucha*)
6 Control of the Senses (*Indriya Nigraha*)
7 Good Intellect/Prudence (*Dhee*)
8 Spiritual Knowledge/Wisdom (*Vidya*)
9 Truthfulness (*Satya*)
10 Absence of Anger (*Akrodha*)

They are sometimes shortened to these five: non-violence, self-restraint, non-stealing, inner purity, truthfulness. Temperance prevents bad karma. We perform these ethical 'duties' with a sense of *pālana* – observing and nourishing. We approach them with *sat bhāvanā* – a truthful attitude, making efforts to serve society through them. The end or purpose is full freedom (*prih*, which is the same word for 'love' in Sanskrit is also 'friend'). The Self (*Paramatman*) is our best friend, outside of our seen and unseen friends (teachers), and the (meditation) mantra which is the inner friend, according to this tradition. The sound of the mantra draws on three universal forces, which we met with earlier:

• *Rajas* – the fire that burns off ignorance (the dynamic principle).
• *Sattva* – the sunlight that nourishes (the pure principle).
• *Tamas* – the moon that brings everything to rest (the principle of inertia).

Patience puts one in the present. *Dhrti* is patience but also firmness, satisfaction, constancy, contentment, and courage to bear with, especially pertinent when we are in any adverse situation and need to control our thoughts, speech, and actions (self-restraint).

Being tolerant of difficulties (endurance) and pardoning wrongs gives space for understanding. *Kshama* is compassion and acceptance of all.

We need to exercise self-control over our senses as the mind is turbulent and can get overstimulated by the external world with all its sights, sounds, and stimuli. The objective here is to find measure in all actions – not too much, not too little (the Golden Mean of Aristotle and the Middle Path of the Buddha).

Not stealing is a little bit different than we might think – it states that we can take only what we need – it's more about what we deserve than what we desire. Here we consider everyone else as equally deserving. The extra we accumulate is theft. Mother Earth and the community as a whole, supply our needs.

Purification cleanses the body–mind. We keep the body, mind, and heart clean through a system (such as Advaita) or a teacher (such as the Shankara-charya). Here we gain a clear understanding of natural law.

With regard to the regulation of the use of the senses, this applies to aspects of measure related to taste as we seek what is refined in our choice of food for the body, mind, and heart.

Spiritual intellect is *buddhi* or reason – it is that use of the intellect which is employed in the search for the causes of things. We are confronted with a choice: to turn to the part, the untruth, and the ego or the whole, the truth, and the Self. Here we decide for the very best.

The Vedas are divine guidance for Self-knowledge and Self-realisation. *Vidya* is the search for natural laws that govern the right relationships between people in society.

Truth is one, indivisible, yet people want their particular brand of truth. The spiritual journey brings one to understand that there is only one Truth.

Anger and agitation block right action. One might have to be tough rather than tender at times, but there is a line demarcating commitment from anger. One must be unattached to the outcome – here we drop the expectation of a result.

Practice

Do we practise patience? Are we forgiving and tolerant of others, of ourselves? Do we aim for moderation in our lives, avoiding excess? Do we take from society more than we need, more than is our due? Would we say we are 'pure in heart', in other words, free from 'evil' in thoughts, words, and deeds? Do we seek balance in activity (measure), mind (reason), and heart (love)? Are we in touch with our higher intelligence, the one that discriminates and discerns wisely and well, ensuring we make good decisions? How much time do we give to reading the words of the wise or Scripture – in serious reflective study? Do we believe and live as if 'all is one' – what actual difference does it make to my life? How often do I get angry/agitated and allow this tyrant of the soul to dominate and overwhelm me? Any serious inner work will require answers to these questions, with the help of the Enneagram, journalling, philosophical ethics, the Ignatian examen, etc.

Ten Universal Principles

American philosopher Robert Spitzer, SJ, outlines ten universal principles by which we can try to make sense of life from a global perspective. They are an attempt to answer the questions: How should I treat others? What can we rely on to guide our actions? How should our laws be framed? What type of society should we seek to build? The following is his list of laws that must govern a reasonable person's thinking and acting (Spitzer, *Ten Universal Principles*, pp. 1–3). I offer them for reflection in our effort to (1) live wisely and well, (2) with and for others, and (3) in just institutions (the threefold aim of what Paul Ricoeur calls his 'little ethics' in *Oneself as Another*):

I   Principles of Reason

Principle 1: The Principle of Complete Explanation (Socrates, Plato, and Aristotle)
The best opinion or theory is the one that explains the most data.
Principle 2: The Principle of Noncontradiction (Plato and Aristotle)
Valid opinions or theories have no internal contradictions.
Classic formulation: A real being cannot both be and not be the same thing, in the same respect, at the same place and time.
Principle 3: The Principle of Objective Evidence (Plato and Aristotle)
Nonarbitrary opinions or theories are based upon publicly verifiable evidence.

II   Principles of Ethics

Principle 4: The Principle of Nonmaleficence (Jesus, Moses, and worldwide religious traditions)
Avoid unnecessary harms; if a harm is unavoidable, minimise it.
Silver Rule: Do *not* do unto others what you would *not* have them do unto you.
Principle 5: The Principle of Consistent Ends and Means (Augustine)
The end does not justify the means.
Principle 6: The Principle of Full Human Potential
Every human being (or group of human beings) deserves to be valued according to the full level of human development, not according to the level of development currently achieved.

III   Principles of Justice and Natural Rights

Principle 7: The Principle of Natural Rights (Suarez, Locke, Jefferson, and Paine)
All human beings possess in themselves (by virtue of their existence alone) the inalienable rights of life, liberty, and property ownership; no government gives these rights, and no government can take them away.
Principle 8: The Principle of the Fundamentality of Rights
(Suarez, Locke, and Jefferson)
The more fundamental right is the one which is necessary for the possibility of the other; where there is a conflict, we should resolve in favour of the fundamental right.
Principle 9: The Principle of Limits to Freedom (Locke and Montesquieu)
One person's (or group's) freedoms cannot impose undue burdens upon other persons (or groups).

IV Fundamental Principle of Identity and Culture

Principle 10: The Principle of Beneficence (Jesus)
Aim at optimal contribution to others and society.
The Golden Rule: Do unto others as you would have them do unto you.

Svadharma

Svadharma is translated as 'duty'. *Dharma*, as we saw earlier, are universal laws of nature. Practising one's *dharma* includes carrying out one's duties and responsibilities – and this is what the ego and the addicted person don't want to hear. It's the opposite of 'easy come, easy go'. *Svadharma* is these laws of nature applied to oneself. It provides *clarity* (we accept personal responsibility for our actions; and if I am driving today, my duty is to drive carefully), *strength* (resilience) and inner understanding as we meet with life's challenges, and it *universalises* our lives, enabling us to see the bigger picture. There is, thus, really no distinction between what is small and what is sacred – everything becomes significant and imbued with love, time, and attention. *Svadharma* raises us up, elevates us, permits us to see ourselves as universal and not just individual beings. We then become of great service to humanity. By doing our duty, we fulfil our destiny. In short, *svadharma* is the shortest route to the Self.

Prayer

This prayer expresses an aspiration of the wise. (That which is in presence cannot be denied. This is a law.)

May all be happy.
May all be without disease (addictions, in particular).
May all creatures have wellbeing, and none be in misery of any sort.
May peace (*Pax*) be everywhere.

Conclusion

We can break the addictive cycle with the help of the Twelve Steps, A.A., contemplative practice (be it Centering Prayer, Christian Meditation, or *Lectio Divina*, to name but three), the Hero's Journey, the Ignatian Examen and *Spiritual Exercises*, the Enneagram, Platonic philosophy, journalling, and *Sanatana Dharma*, transitioning from autopilot, where we are asleep at the helm/ wheel, to being fully awake here and now: from stagnation to growth, from compulsion to release, from fixation to freedom, and from addicted to liberated humanity – the land of pure peace as ultimate promise.

Postscript

Mimetic Desire

I would like to pose one final question for consideration: what is the addicted person's desire? Moreover, what is anyone's desire? René Girard's (1923–2015) anthropological analysis of mimetic desire can shed much light on addiction in its relation to desire. The work of this French theorist is relevant to our foregoing discussion. Here, I simply want to offer a few brief Girardian reflections on mimetic desire in connection with addiction.

Imitation (*mimesis*), which is the highest form of flattery, centres on 'models' – people or things that show us what is worth wanting and around which or whom our social lives revolve. Collective models include the media, movies, and the proliferation of advertising messages which bombard us daily. Mimetic desire draws us to things. The lie is that of the individual subject making autonomous life choices. The truth is that our deepest desires are mediated by others. Our desires are generated and shaped by models. This creates a cycle of rivalry. We can't blame our backgrounds or parents or our education, class, or country. The enemy is us! The obstacle/uninvited guest to this party is the mimetic rival whom *we* are copying. There's always somebody who's richer, slimmer, better. Unconsciously imitating them sets up mimetic futility. Mimetic desire is a persuasive and powerful social contagion which contributes to addiction (see Girard, 'Eating Disorders and Mimetic Desire', available online; and *I See Satan Fall Like Lightening*). Addiction, so, for Girard means that the subject does not stand free toward the object but, rather, that the subject is addicted to the object in so far as it is mediated by the mimetic model.

One might ask where do we get our desires from? The answer is other models. (In the Garden of Eden, Eve had no initial desire to eat the fruit from the forbidden tree until the Serpent suggested a desire to her.) We see what we want in a refracted light. Desire is always desire of the Other. We are born imitators; we want what others want simply because they want it. Desire creates conflict – rivalry, violence. (Recent work in mirror neurons has contributed to the

DOI: 10.4324/9781003422570-13

neurological understanding of imitation.) I may desire an addictive or forbidden substance because my desire increases when it is denied. Behind my desire for this particular thing, which all these others desire too, is my real desire for being, which Girard calls *metaphysical* desire. So desire is mimetic and metaphysical. It is not of this world. That's why nothing finite – no line of coke or endless cavorting or consumption – can satiate the heart's true desire. We exist in layers of mimetic desire. Furthermore, mimetic desire is socially contagious – it spreads like wildfire. Everyone gets caught up in it. There is the social dimension which must be taken into account.

When a mimetic crisis occurs, society expels or eliminates one person or group of people – Jews, Catholics, etc. The scapegoat provides an outlet for their violence (the mimetic mob). Envy is the engine of destructive and dangerous mimetic desire. In our search to be satisfied, our desires proliferate. Desire is metonymical in that it creates more desire, as desire springs from lack and so the addicted subject – every one of us – is embroiled in a perpetual quest for more and more with the forlorn hope that something will finally fulfil. What to do? We can live inauthentically through an unintentionally mimetic life or try to transform our desires, from thin to thick desires, for example, by doing the one thing we are destined to do, on which we would stake our life or simply this: just wanting what we already have (see *Wanting* by Luke Burgis).

This is not easy because where there is *mimesis* there is also what Martin Heidegger calls *Mitsein*, that is to say, other people. My being is alongside others. Being is being *with*. Such is the inter-individuality of existence. *Mimesis* is a modus of *Mitsein*. I live exactly like 'they' live, in the like manner of the 'They' (*das Man*). One becomes addicted to the choices and preferences and objects of the They, of which I am a part (not apart from). My existence is shared, mutual, intertwined with all those others. If the notion of a solitary self is false, the real truth is our shared sociality. We are so far from being independent, sovereign, and atomistic; rather, we are utterly absorbed in the world, existing alongside other entities with their brazenly borrowed and bold desires. I am immersed in the They, in what Lacan calls the Symbolic Order. (This is why a political philosophy needs to be articulated which is based not on the neo-liberal fantasy of the autonomous individual pursuing his pleasure and preferences in a vacuum but on some communitarian vision of the common good.)

Addiction has, thus, a triangular structure: me, the object, and the model. We are drawn to what others want; two desires converge on objects. Desire is social. My desires neither originate from an attractive object nor from an authentic subject but are always mediated by a model. I desire precisely because others desire. This means that *addiction is grounded in mimesis*, which is the glue of society. Can we escape the mechanisms of mass and massive *mimesis*? Perhaps not. But we can transform desire even if it can't be entirely transcended; we can name our models; we can begin to stop chasing after things we don't truly want; we can discover our deepest desires; we can realise our mimetic acts; we can even perhaps gaze on the face of the Other (to draw on Emmanuel Levinas) and love them from a place of distance. To do so, we will have to go down to the root of our desire to tear the energy from its object. Isn't the work of such purification, as Simone Weil taught, ultimately the separation of good from covetousness?

Bibliography

Alcoholics Anonymous, fourth edition. Alcoholics Anonymous World Services, Inc., New York, 2001.

Almaas, A. H. *Keys to the Enneagram*. Shambhala, Colorado, 2021.

American Psychiatric Association. *Diagnostic and Statistical Manual of Mental Disorders*, fifth edition. American Psychiatric Publishing, San Francisco, 2013.

Benedict, Saint. *The Rule of St. Benedict in English*. Ed. Timothy Fry. The Liturgical Press, Minnesota, 1982.

Bianchi, Enzo. *Lectio Divina*. SPCK, London, 2008.

Blonna, Richard. *Coping with Stress in a Changing World*. McGraw-Hill, Chicago, 2011.

Bourgeault, Cynthia. *Centering Prayer and Inner Awakening*. Cowley Publications, Plymouth, 2004.

Bourgeault, Cynthia. *The Heart of Centering Prayer: Nondual Christianity in Theory and Practice*. Shambhala, Boulder, 2016.

Bowlby, John. *Attachment and Loss*, vols. 1–3. Pimlico, London, 1997.

Burgis, Luke. *Wanting: The Power of Mimetic Desire, and How to Want What You Need*. Swift, London, 2021.

Campbell, Joseph. *The Hero with a Thousand Faces*. Fontana Press, London, 1993.

Campbell, Joseph (with Bill Moyers). *The Power of Myth*. Anchor Books, New York, 1991.

Chestnut, Beatrice. *The Complete Enneagram*. She Writes Press, Berkeley, 2013.

Costello, Stephen. *Applied Logotherapy: Viktor Frankl's Philosophical Psychology*. Cambridge Scholars Publishing, Newcastle Upon Tyne, 2019.

Costello, Stephen J. *Between Speech and Silence: From Communicating to Meditating*. Pickwick Publications, Oregon, 2022a.

Costello, Stephen J. *Dynamics of Discernment: A Guide to Good Decision-Making*. Pickwick Publications, Oregon, 2022b.

Costello, Stephen J. *The Nine Faces of Fear: Ego, Enneatype, Essence*. Pickwick Publications, Oregon, 2022c.

Daniels, David. *The Essential Enneagram*. HarperOne, San Francisco, 2009.

Fabry, Joseph (ed.). *Logotherapy in Action*. Jason Aronson, New York and London, 1979.

Ferry, Luc. *The Wisdom of the Myths*. Harper Perennial, New York, London, and Toronto, 2014.

Ficino, Masrsilio. *Gardens of Philosophy*. Trans. Arthur Farndell. Shepheard-Walwyn Publishers, London, 2006.

Frankl, Viktor. *Man's Search for Meaning*. Rider, London-Sydney-Auckland-Johannesburg, 2001.

Frankl, Viktor. *On the Theory and Therapy of Mental Disorders*. Trans. James DuBois. Brunner-Routledge, New York and Hove, 2004.

Freud, Anna. *The Ego and the Mechanisms of Defence*. Routledge, London, 1992.

Freud, Sigmund. *Civilization and Its Discontents*. The Hogarth Press, London, 1982.

Girard, René. *I See Satan Fall Like Lightening*. Trans. James Williams. Orbis Books, New York, 2001.

Girard, René. 'Eating Disorders and Mimetic Desire'. https://doi.org/10.1007/s11013-018-9574-y. (Originally in *Culture, Medicine, and Psychiatry* 42, 2018, 552–583.)

Goeders, Nick E. 'The Impact of Stress on Addiction', *European Neuropsychopharmacology* 13 (6), 2003, 435–441.

Green, Jim. *Meditation and Addiction*. Meditatio – an outreach of The World Community for Christian Tradition, UK, 2012.

Hederman, Mark Patrick. *Living the Mystery: What Lies Between Science and Religion*. Columba Press, Dublin, 2019.

Jenner K. *The Enneagram for Recovery*. Happy Destiny Publishing, 2020.

Jung, C. G. *Letters*, vol. 2, 1951–1961. Eds. G. Adler and A. Jaffe. Trans. R. F. Hull. Princeton University Press, New York, 1975.

Jung, C. G. *Psychology and Alchemy*. Collected Works of C.G. Jung, vol. 12. Routledge, London, 1980.

Jung, C. G. *The Practice of Psychotherapy*. Collected Works of C.G. Jung, vol. 16. Princeton University Press, New Jersey, 1982.

Keating, Thomas. *Open Mind, Open Heart*. Bloomsbury Continuum, London, 2006.

Keating, Thomas. *The Heart of the World: An Introduction to Contemplative Christianity*. Crossroad Publishing, New York, 2008 (1981).

Keating, Thomas. *Divine Therapy and Addiction: Centering Prayer and the Twelve Steps*. Lantern Books, Brooklyn, 2011a.

Keating, Thomas. *Invitation to Love: The Way of Christian Contemplation*. Bloomsbury, London, 2011b.

Keating, Thomas. *Consenting to God As God Is*. Lantern Publishing, New York, 2020a.

Keating, Thomas. *Intimacy with God: An Introduction to Centering Prayer*. Crossroad Publishing, New York, 2020b.

Kumar, Satish. *Spiritual Compass: The Three Qualities of Life*. Green Books, Cambridge, 2007.

Liquorman, Wayne. *The Power of Powerlessness: Advaita and the 12 Steps of Recovery*. Advaita Press, California, 2012.

Maddi, Salvatore, and Khoshaba, Deborah M. *Resilience at Work*. Amacom, New York, 2005.

Main, John. *The Inner Christ*. Darton, Longman and Todd, London, 1980.

Main, John. *Word into Silence: A Manual for Christian Meditation*. Canterbury Press, London, 2019 (1980).

Maté, Gabor. *In the Realm of Hungry Ghosts: Close Encounters with Addiction*. North Atlantic Books, Berkeley, 2010.

May, Gerald. *Grace and Addiction*. Harper Collins, New York, 1991a.

May, Rollo. *The Cry for Myth*. W.W. Norton & Company, London and New York, 1991b.

McCabe, Ian. *Carl Jung and Alcoholics Anonymous*. Routledge, London and New York, 2015.

Naifeh, Sam. 'Archetypal Foundation of Addiction and Recovery', *Journal of Analytical Psychology* 40, 1995, 133–159.

Pieper, Josef. *A Brief Reader on the Virtues of the Human Heart*. Ignatius Press, San Francisco, 1991 (1988).

Plato. *The Republic*. Trans. Desmond Lee. Penguin Books, London, 1974.

Plato. *Complete Works*. Hackett Publishing, Indianapolis/Cambridge, 1997.

Redfearn, Joseph. *My Self, My Many Selves*. Routledge, London, 1994.

Ricoeur, Paul. *Oneself As Another*. Trans. Kathleen Blamey. University of Chicago Press, 1995.

Riso, Don and Hudson, Russ. *The Wisdom of the Enneagram*. Bantam Books, London, New York, and Toronto, 1999.

Rohr, Richard. *Breathing Under Water*: *Spirituality and the Twelve Steps*. Franciscan Media, Ohio, 2011.

Saraswatī, Sri Shāntānanda. *Good Company*: *An Anthology*. The Study Society, London, 2017.

Schoen, David. *The War of the Gods in Addiction*. Spring Journal Books, New Orleans, 2009.

Selhub, Eva. *Resilience for Dummies*. John Wiley & Sons, New York, 2021.

Spitzer, Robert. *Ten Universal Principles*: *A Brief Philosophy of the Life Issues*. Ignatius Press, San Francisco, 2009.

Sponville, André-Comte. *A Short Treatise on the Great Virtues*. William Heinemann, London, 2002.

Stabile, Suzanne. *The Journey Toward Wholeness*. Intervarsity Press, Illinois, 2021.

Thomas, Alexander and Chess, Stella. *Temperament and Development*. Brunner/Mazel, New York, 1977.

Thompson, Damian. *The Fix: How Addiction is Invading Our Lives and Taking Over Our World*. Collins, London, 2013.

Urick, E. J. *The Platonic Quest*. Concord Grove Press, California, 1983.

Vaillant, George Eman. *Adaptation to Life*. Little Brown, Boston, 1977.

Vaillant, George Eman. *The Natural History of Alcoholism*. Harvard University Press, Cambridge, Massachusetts, 1995.

Vogler, Christopher. *The Writer's Journey*. Michael Wise Productions, California, 2007.

Watson, William M. *Sacred Story: An Ignatian Examen for the Third Millennium*. The Sacred Story Institute, Washington, DC, 2012.

World Health Organisation. *International Classification of Diseases*, tenth edition. World Health Organisation, Geneva, 1992.

Zoja, Luigi. *Drugs, Alcohol, and Initiation: The Modern Search for Ritual*. Sugo, Boston, 1989.

Index

For Product Safety Concerns and Information please contact our EU
representative GPSR@taylorandfrancis.com
Taylor & Francis Verlag GmbH, Kaufingerstraße 24, 80331 München, Germany

www.ingramcontent.com/pod-product-compliance
Lightning Source LLC
Chambersburg PA
CBHW050613280326
41932CB00016B/3027